Chronic Illness in Children

An Evidence-Based Approach

Laura L. Hayman, PhD, RN, FAAN, is a Professor in the Division of Nursing, The Steinhardt School of Education, New York University and Adjunct Professor, Integrative and Behavioral Cardiovascular Health Program, Mount Sinai School of Medicine, New York. Dr. Hayman received her MSN in Nursing of Children and PhD in Interdisciplinary Studies in Human Development from the University of Pennsylvania. She was a member of the University of Pennsylvania faculty (in Nursing and later Medicine) for nearly 20 years, and served as Chair of the Nursing of Children Division. Following this, she was the Carl W. and Margaret Davis Walter Professor of Nursing at Case Western Reserve University. Her research focuses on primary prevention of cardiovascular disease (CVD) and includes a twelve-year study of genetic and environmental determinants of risk factors for CVD in twins as they advance through childhood and adolescence. Dr. Hayman is a Fellow in the American Academy of Nursing, the American Heart Association, and the Society of Behavioral Medicine. She has co-edited five previous books and has served on numerous expert panels and editorial boards, including (currently) *American Journal of Health Behavior, MCN: The Journal of Maternal-Child Nursing*, and *Annals of Behavioral Medicine*.

Margaret M. Mahon, PhD, RN, FAAN, is Clinical Nurse Specialist, End-of-Life Care, Hospital of the University of Pennsylvania, and Senior Fellow, Center for Bioethics, University of Pennsylvania School of Medicine. Dr. Mahon's major research has focused on children's concepts of death, bereaved siblings, and bereaved parents' experiences and responses. Her clinical experience with children and families includes advanced practice nursing roles in pediatric trauma, intensive care, and chronic illness. Dr. Mahon has worked with bereaved children and families in hospital, hospice, home, school, and other community settings. She hosts the "Kid's Corner" radio program designed to provide parents, teachers, and children with information and counsel on issues in child and family health care. Dr. Mahon is a Fellow of the American Academy of Nursing.

J. Rick Turner, PhD, is an experimental psychologist who has spent 15 years conducting research in the field of Cardiovascular Behavioral Medicine. His research has focused on the effects of stress on the cardiovascular system, and the possible role of stress-induced responses in the development of cardiovascular disease. He has published 50 scientific papers describing his collaborative research, two textbooks, and two previous edited volumes. His authored text entitled *Cardiovascular Reactivity and Stress: Patterns of Physiological Response* (New York: 1994) introduced the research methodology and findings of cardiovascular reactivity research to undergraduate and graduate students. Dr. Turner has received research awards from the Society for Psychophysiological Research and the American Psychosomatic Society. He is Founding Editor of the Sage Publications Series in Behavioral Medicine and Health Psychology, and a Fellow of the Society of Behavioral Medicine. He lives in Chapel Hill, North Carolina, where he works as a Medical Editor in the pharmaceutical industry.

Chronic Illness in Children

An Evidence-Based Approach

Laura L. Hayman, PhD, RN, FAAN
Margaret M. Mahon, PhD, CRNP, FAAN
J. Rick Turner, PhD
Editors

 Springer Publishing Company

Springer Publishing Company, Inc.
536 Broadway
New York, NY 10012-3955

Acquisitions Editor: Ruth Chasek
Production Editor: Jeanne W. Libby
Cover design by Joanne E. Honigman

01 02 03 04 05/5 4 3 2 1

Library of Congress Cataloging-in-Publication Data

Chronic illness in children : an evidence-based approach / [edited by] Laura L. Hayman, Margaret M. Mahon, J. Rick Turner.
    p. ; cm.
  Includes bibliographical references and index.
  ISBN 0-8261-3856-X
  1. Chronic diseases in children. 2. Chronically ill children.
3. Evidence-based medicine. I. Hayman, Laura Lucia. II. Mahon, Margaret M. III. Turner, J. Rick.
  [DNLM: 1. Chronic Disease—Child. 2. Evidence-Based Medicine—methods—Child.
WS 200 C55763 2002]
RJ380 .C5875 2002
618.92—dc21

                                  2002070498
                                      CIP

Printed in the United States of America by Maple-Vail.

Contents

Contributors

Patricia V. Burkhart, PhD, RN
Assistant Professor
University of Kentucky
School of Nursing
Lexington, Kentucky

Harry Davis, MS
Medical College of Georgia
Georgia Prevention Institute
Augusta, Georgia

Jacqueline Dunbar-Jacob, PhD, RN, FAAN
Professor & Dean
University of Pittsburgh
School of Nursing
Pittsburgh, Pennsylvania

Romy C. Engel, PhD
Ferkauf Graduate School
Yeshiva University
Bronx, New York

Diane Carol Hudson-Barr, PhD, RN
Clinical Nurse Specialist, Brenner Children's Hospital
Wake Forest University Baptist Medical Center
Winston-Salem, North Carolina

Janet Johnston, MSN, CPNP
Assistant Professor
Pediatric Pulmonary Center
Department of Pediatric Pulmonary, School of Medicine
Affiliate Faculty, School of Nursing
University of Alabama at Birmingham
Birmingham, Alabama

Sally A. Lambert, PhD, RN
Clinical Nurse Specialist
Rainbow Babies & Children's Hospital
University Hospitals of Cleveland
Cleveland, Ohio

Terri H. Lipman, PhD, CRNP, FAAN
Associate Professor, Nursing of Children Division
University of Pennsylvania
School of Nursing
Pediatric Nurse Practitioner
Division of Endocrinology & Diabetes
The Children's Hospital of Philadelphia
Philadelphia, Pennsylvania

Barbara G. Melamed, PhD
Professor, Division of Social & Behavioral Sciences
Mercy College
Dobbs Ferry, New York

Ida M. (Ki) Moore, DNS, FAAN
Professor & Director of the Nursing Practice Division
College of Nursing
University of Arizona
Tucson, Arizona

Margaret P. Shepard, PhD, RN
Director of Graduate Studies
Temple University
School of Nursing
Philadelphia, Pennsylvania

Frank A. Treiber, PhD
Professor of Pediatrics & Psychology
Medical College of Georgia
Georgia Prevention Institute
Augusta, Georgia

Anne Turner-Henson, DSN, RN
Associate Professor, University of Alabama School of Nursing
University of Alabama at Birmingham
Birmingham, Alabama

Introduction

The experience of chronic illness poses unique and complex challenges for children, their families, health care providers, and systems of health care delivery. Evidence-based health care, in this context, is designed to provide effective interventions that optimize health and developmental outcomes for children with chronic conditions. Toward this goal, this text addresses the state-of-the science, current practice, emerging issues and research directions relevant to selected chronic childhood conditions. Conceptualized within a developmental-systems framework, emphasis is placed on the child and the "contexts of care" including the family, school, and community. Across content areas, health is viewed as more than the absence of disease, with emphasis on physical, psychosocial, cognitive, and emotional functioning. Relatedly, evidence-based interventions are offered with the ultimate goal of maximizing the child's opportunities for health.

In chapter 1 of this text, Anne Turner-Henson and Janet Johnston, advanced practice nurse specialists, illustrate the challenges and opportunities in providing evidence-based care for children with asthma. In describing asthma as the "single largest public health burden in pediatrics," these authors identify both individual and population-based approaches to prevention and management of this highly prevalent chronic condition. Recent advances in pharmacologic and self-care therapies are outlined with emphasis on physiological, behavioral, and parent/family factors that have the potential to influence health behaviors and health outcomes for children and youth with asthma. Similarly, in chapter 2, Terri Lipman, nurse researcher and expert clinician, presents an overview of the epidemiology and multifactorial etiology of type 1 diabetes in children and youth. Emphasis is placed on both genetic and environmental influences on the development and expression of diabetes in childhood, individual and population-based prevention strategies, and multidisciplinary approaches to diabetes management. In chapter 3, expert nurse clinicians and researchers Diane Hudson-Barr and Sally Lambert describe the six current categories of Juvenile Idiopathic Arthritis (JIA) and the related scientific advances that have resulted in this new classification scheme. As in other chronic conditions discussed in this text, the goal of interventions is on early and continuing recognition of the impact of JIA on the child's physical, psychosocial, cognitive and emotional functioning, the daily activities and quality of family life, and multidisciplinary approaches to management. As described by Hudson-Barr and Lambert, chronic pain is a major component of symptom management and holistic care for children with JIA. Developmentally appropriate assessment strategies are essential for optimal pharmacologic and multimodal management of chronic pain in children and youth with JIA.

The past decade has witnessed substantial advances in our understanding of the biological basis of childhood cancer, methods of detection and diagnosis, and multimodal therapies. In chapter 4, Ida (Ki) Moore, expert clinician and researcher, details these advances, results of her seminal research on cognitive and psychosocial late effects, and offers evidence-based interventions designed to improve the quality of life for survivors of childhood cancer.

Cardiovascular disease (CVD) remains the leading cause of morbidity and premature mortality in the United States. In chapter 5, Frank Treiber and colleagues describe the early childhood origins of CVD and suggest exaggerated cardiovascular responsivity (CVR) to stress as a candidate risk factor. A biobehavioral model of CVR is presented as a possible mechanism leading to overt manifestation of CVD via ventricular and vascular remodeling. Implications for primary prevention of CVD are offered, based on available evidence and focused on behavioral approaches to lowering blood pressure in hypertensive children and youth.

Section II of this text emphasizes topics relevant to clinicians and scholars from the many disciplines that care for children with chronic conditions or conduct research focused on chronically ill children and their families. Chapter 6 presents a state-of-the-art and science overview highlighting the central and essential role of the family in chronic childhood illness. Margaret Shepard and Margaret Mahon, expert child-family researchers and clinicians, provide the evidence to guide family-focused interventions applicable across childhood chronic illness. As suggested throughout this text, the family is viewed as the most important context of care for children.

Throughout the diagnostic and treatment phases of chronic illness, an important part of caring for children is appraisal of stress and enhancement of effective coping mechanisms. In chapter 7, psychologists Romy Engel and Barbara Melamed emphasize developmental processes as a critical component of children's appraisal of stress and coping responses. They also provide an evidence-based model that highlights developmental tasks as part of intervention strategies for children's coping.

Adherence, the extent to which individuals/patients comply with a prescribed therapeutic regimen, is now recognized across disciplines as a multilevel challenge involving the patient (chronically ill child), provider, and system of health care delivery. In childhood chronic illness, lack of adherence to recommended treatments has significant implications for health and developmental outcomes. In chapter 8, adherence researchers Patricia Burkhart and Jacqueline Dunbar-Jacob present a comprehensive review of this research in children and youth, emphasize developmental processes as a critical determinant of adherence behavior, and define directions for future research focused on multicomponent preventive-interventions.

Within the context of 21st century health care, the experience of chronic illness continues to pose unique and complex challenges for children and their families. Maximizing the child's opportunities for health is a goal shared by child health care professionals, educators, and advocates. Toward this goal, this volume was created for child health care professionals and students from many disciplines who care for chronically ill children and their families.

PART I

Major Chronic Diseases: Epidemiology, Etiology, and Management

CHAPTER 1

Pediatric Asthma

Anne Turner-Henson and Janet Johnston

Asthma is the single, largest public health burden in pediatrics. During childhood and adolescence, pediatric asthma can have a profound impact on growth and development, and on the daily lives of families. Over the past few decades, assessment, management, and self-care strategies for children and adolescents with asthma and chronic pulmonary disorders have resulted in increased longevity, along with increased shift from hospital to home care. Significant advances in pharmacologic products and durable medical equipment have resulted in improved disease outcomes and quality of life for these children and their families. The goal of this chapter is not only to describe the current pharmacological and self-care therapies for children and adolescents with asthma, but also to identify what physiological, behavioral, or parent factors influence the health promoting behaviors for these children and adolescents. By identifying behaviors that are health promoting and those that are not, this chapter provides a scientific knowledge base upon which health professionals may build behavioral strategies and clinical interventions to promote the wellness of children and adolescents with asthma.

OVERVIEW OF EPIDEMIOLOGY

Approximately 8 million children in the U.S. have asthma (ALA, 2001), with increased prevalence in minorities, particularly blacks and inner city children (Gergen, Fowler, Maurer, Davis, & Overpeck, 1998). While the prevalence of asthma is greater in minorities, greater frequencies of asthma are seen in males, children living in poverty, and children from inner cities (Newacheck & Halfon, 1998).

Pediatric asthma morbidity has steadily increased over the past decade. Increased asthma morbidity has been particularly noted in young children (< 5 years) with a two- to threefold increase in morbidity in African American children. Asthma morbidity has resulted in 7.3 million days of restricted bed rest, 10.1 million days missed from school, 12.9 million contacts with physicians, and 200,000 hospitalizations per year. As compared to children without asthma, children with asthma use substantially more health care services: 3.1 times as many prescriptions, 1.9 times more ambulatory care visits, 2.2 times more emergency department visits, and 3.5 times as many hospitalizations (Lozano, Sullivan, Smith, & Weiss, 1999). The impact of childhood asthma on families' budgets results in the largest single indirect cost of asthma. This cost approached $4.64 billion in 1994, largely due to children's school absences that resulted in reduced parental employment productivity (Weiss, Sullivan, & Lyttle, 2000). Pediatric asthma is the leading cause of school absenteeism and ranks first among childhood chronic conditions in limiting activities of daily living (Newacheck, Budetti, & Halfon, 1986).

Disparities in social position play a large role in the racial differences in pediatric asthma prevalence and its resulting morbidity and mortality. Minority populations, specifically those from lower socioeconomic and urban, inner city areas have increased asthma rates and greater asthma morbidity and mortality. While black children have increased asthma prevalence (blacks– 7.2% as compared with 3% in whites) (Eggleston, 1998), black adolescents are more likely to have poorly controlled asthma (Murray, Stang, & Tierney, 1997). Black children are more likely to experience greater restrictions in activity, and to report more severe functional disability (Newacheck & Halfon, 1998). In addition, black children are disproportionately less likely to use preventive services for asthma care (Lozano, Connell, & Koepsell, 1995) and do rely more often on emergency department and inpatient services for asthma care.

DISEASE PROCESS IN ASTHMA

Asthma is characterized as a chronic inflammatory disease of the airways, with episodic symptoms. Asthma results from complex interactions among inflammatory cells, mediators, and the cells and tissues that reside in the airways. In particular, mast cells, eosinophil, T lymphocytes, neutrophils, and epithelial cells play a role in this chronic inflammatory disease. Inflammation in asthma causes recurrent episodes of wheezing, breathlessness, chest tightness, and cough (particularly at night and early morning). These episodes are associated with airway flow obstruction that is usually reversible either spontaneously or with treatment. Airway inflammation also causes bronchial hyperresponsiveness to a variety of stimuli.

The development of pediatric asthma has been strongly linked to the sensitization of airways. Causal risk factors in pediatric asthma sensitize the airways and result in the onset of asthma. Atopy, the genetic predisposition for developing an IgE mediated response to common aeroallergens, is the strongest identifiable predisposing factor in the development of asthma in children. Allergens may cause the onset of asthma by continuously stimulating chronic allergic inflammation of the airways. Clinical studies are now exploring the relationship between allergen exposure and sensitization in young children (Landau, 1996). While not firmly established, the risk of sensitization to allergens may peak during the first year of life, when exposure occurs in conjunction with the ongoing development of the mucosal immune system.

Several factors have been hypothesized to increase the risk for the development of asthma including genetic, gender, intrauterine environment, preterm delivery, and other environmental factors (Landau, 1996). It has been suggested that 30–40% of the population are at risk for asthma or atopy; and genetic markers on chromosomes 5, 11, and 14 have been associated with asthma and atopy (LeSouef, 1997). Lower pulmonary flow rates in males from birth to early adolescence suggest that males have smaller airways and increased muscle tone, providing evidence to support the physiological basis for the increasing prevalence of asthma in males (Landau, 1996).

Maternal smoking during pregnancy and preterm delivery have also been associated with asthma. Environmental exposure to allergens and other substances, particularly inhaled substances (Institute of Medicine, 2000), is clearly associated with the exacerbations of asthma, though the causal relationship to the development of asthma is less well understood (Landau, 1996). Sensitization to common allergens, particularly pollens, is greater for those residing in urban areas. It has been suggested that air pollution may make pollens more allergenic or may cause damage to the respiratory epithelial mucosa, thus allowing easier access of allergens to the antigen-presenting cells. Children who spend long periods of time outside and those in crowded urban areas have greater risks for developing asthma, probably due to the increase environmental exposure to poor indoor and outdoor air quality, and high concentrations of house dust mite, molds, and cockroach antigen. While passive smoke has been clearly linked with increased risks for acute respiratory disease and asthma morbidity, it has not been found to be a causative agent for asthma.

ASTHMA ASSESSMENT AND MANAGEMENT

The National Heart, Lung, and Blood Institute (NHLBI) of the National Institutes of Health (1997a, 1997b) released guidelines for the diagnosis and management of asthma. These guidelines provided updated diagnostic categories and recommendations for the pharmacologic treatment focusing on the inflammatory responses of asthma. Pediatric-specific asthma management guidelines have been published by the American Academy of Asthma, Allergy and Immunology (AAAAI, 1999), focusing on child- and adolescent-specific asthma management strategies. Goals of pediatric asthma care should include: prevention of chronic and troublesome symptoms, maintenance of normal pulmonary function, maintenance of normal daily activity, prevention of recurrent exacerbations of asthma, provision for optimal pharmacotherapy with minimal adverse effects, and meeting families' expectations for asthma care.

Classification of asthma is based on symptom frequency, nighttime symptoms, exacerbation character and frequency, and lung function variability prior to treatment. Diagnostic categories include: mild intermittent, mild persistent, moderate persistent, and severe persistent. Table 1.1 provides an overview of the diagnostic categories, symptom frequency, and pharmacological strategies including both long and short-term measures. Coupled with pharmacological treatment, primary prevention strategies focus primarily on environmental control of triggers. Control of environmental triggers and primary prevention will be discussed in the later section of this chapter.

CHILDHOOD FACTORS IN ASTHMA

Effective asthma management results in children with active lifestyles, both at home and school, as well as those who enjoy uninterrupted sleep from asthma symptoms. However, attainment of this goal requires special attention to children's unique physiological states (different from the adult), growth and development, and maturing self-care abilities in light of the tasks of effective asthma management. The tasks of effective asthma management include: (1) daily monitoring of asthma symptoms and responding to changes in symptoms based on an individualized asthma management plan, (2) daily medication administration (except for those with mild, intermittent asthma who require medication only as needed for symptom management), and (3) adjustments in the environment to avoid or reduce exposure to specific asthma triggers or allergens that excite an acute asthma episode. Additionally, these

TABLE 1.1 Asthma Diagnostic Categories, Symptoms, and Pharmacologic Management

Diagnostic category	Symptoms		General comments	Pharmacologic long-term measures	Pharmacologic short-term measures
	Daytime	Nighttime			
Mild Intermittent	≤ 2 times/week	≤ 2 times/ month	Normal pulmonary measures Intensity of episodes will vary Symptoms usually seen with upper respiratory infections or sustained physical activity	No daily medications needed	Short-acting inhaled beta$_2$ agonist for symptoms
Mild Persistent	3–6 times/week	3–4 times/ month	May affect activity	Daily medications: Antiinflammatory either inhaled corticosteroid (low dose), cromolyn, or nedocromil. Leukotriene modifiers may be considered (for children 2 yrs and older), although their position in therapy is not fully established.	Short-acting inhaled beta$_2$ agonist for symptoms

(continued)

TABLE 1.1 *(continued)*

Diagnostic category	Symptoms		Pharmacologic long-term measures	Pharmacologic short-term measures
	Daytime	Nighttime	General comments	
Moderate Persistent	Daily	≥ 5 times/month	Episodes may affect activity	Daily medications: antiinflammatory inhaled corticosteroids (medium dose) and long-acting bronchodilators or leukotriene modifiers (oral medication)	Short-acting inhaled beta₂ agonist for symptoms
Severe Persistent	Continual	Frequent	Frequent episodes Limited physical activity	Daily medications: antiinflammatory inhaled corticosteroids (high dose) and long-acting bronchodilator and oral corticosteroids	Short-acting inhaled beta₂ agonist for symptoms

(AAAAI, 1999; NHLBI, 1997a)

*An individual's classification may change over time.

*Children at any level of severity of asthma can have mild, moderate, or severe exacerbations of asthma. Some children with intermittent asthma may experience severe or life-threatening episodes separated by long periods of normal lung function and no symptoms.

*Children with 2 or more asthma episodes per week (i.e., progressively worsening symptoms that may last hours or days) tend to have moderate to severe persistent asthma.

tasks must also be continued while in other environments, such as the school or recreational activity settings.

Monitoring and Assessment

Monitoring and assessment of asthma status (e.g., symptoms, medication use, etc.) is an essential component of pediatric asthma care. Prompt recognition and treatment of changes in asthma status will often provide earlier reversal of changes in the airways.

Self-care management in children and adolescents is dependent upon the individual's cognitive abilities, maturity, and fine/gross motor physical skills to manage the daily responsibilities of asthma care. The cognitive and language ability of the child will affect how well the child is able to perceive and communicate changes in breathing patterns. Both the parent and child should assess daily for asthma symptoms such as increased cough, wheezing, shortness of breath, or irritability, then initiate additional therapy as instructed. Beginning in the preschool years, the child should be instructed in recognizing changes in breathing and communicating this to the responsible adult. Being able to recognize who the responsible adult is in a situation should be practiced with a preschool child. Responsibility for recognizing changes in breathing patterns, communicating these changes, and initiating additional therapies in asthma status should increase as the child matures and demonstrates appropriate ability to assess and monitor his or her own health status. Maturity of the individual will vary, though starting in the preschool years with parental supervision, children should be encouraged to begin to accept responsibility for selected self-care activities.

Fine/gross motor abilities of children and adolescents also play a role in these assessment and self-care management strategies. For example, two components in assessment of pulmonary function is spirometry and peak flow measures. These maneuvers require fine/gross motor skills. Both require the individual follow verbal instructions closely, hold the mouthpiece without air leakage, then fully inhale and exhale. Incorrect technique in these assessments can lead to misguided prescriptions or management plans. Children < 7 years old generally lack the fine/gross motor skills to perform these measures. Therefore, assessment of pulmonary function must rely on other measures such as parent or child recall of symptom history, auscultation of lung fields, assessment of respiratory effort, or pulse oximetry.

Medication Administration

Asthma medications include both long-term controller (also known as *preventive*) medications (typically inhaled corticosteroids) that reduce and prevent chronic inflammation, as well as quick relief medication that reduce the acute symptoms of asthma (i.e., cough, wheeze, chest tightness). There is also growing research interest in the possibility that early treatment with inhaled corticosteroids may prevent airway remodeling and the development of irreversible structural changes in the airway of the child. For both the benefit of an active, healthy life with minimal symptoms and the possibility of avoiding permanent airway changes, daily medications are recommended for all children with persistent asthma.

Persistent asthma is a chronic condition that requires daily medication. This is often difficult to achieve when parents and the child perceive asthma as an episodic condition. Poor control is most noticeable as the child's activity increases. Therefore, children and families often limit activities and modify their lifestyles to control asthma symptoms, rather than use adequate medication to control airway inflammation.

Preventive medications (e.g., inhaled cortiocosteriods) for asthma do not immediately relieve symptoms, but require faithful use over time to benefit the individual's perception of asthma control. This may further support the parent or child's tendency to omit the medications when the asthma status is stable and without symptoms. Inadequate medication administration may also reinforce the child's or parent's perception that preventive medications are ineffective and not necessary, and may result in poor adherence to the asthma medication plan.

Many of the asthma medications are inhaled. Skills required to properly use a metered dose inhaler are difficult to perform, especially for a child < 7 years of age. Poor technique in medication administration will result in improper medication deposition, thus leading to acute asthma episodes or an increase in chronic symptoms. Spacers (holding chambers with mouthpiece or face mask, that ensure that aerosol particles have a slower velocity and a smaller particle size when they reach the airway) as well as nebulized medications, are available to improve deposition of medication.

Fine/gross motor skills used with inhaled medications should be taught and frequently assessed (with return demonstration by the child) by the health care provider with each office visit and reinforced by the parents in the home. Various products are available to best match the development and skills of the child. Newer inhalant delivery devices, such as dry powdered inhalers, are currently being investigated. In addition, the child and family should be intimately involved in decision making about therapeutic issues such as medication choice and method of medication delivery and frequency.

Lifestyle and Environmental Controls

Children with asthma and their families will attain better asthma control by making adjustments to their lifestyles or environments to eliminate or reduce the child's exposure to common allergens or irritants that provoke asthma. Families are commonly asked to institute measures to reduce dust mite exposure (encase bedding, wash linens frequently in hot water, dust/mop weekly), remove animals from the home, eliminate roaches and mold from the home. Irritants such as smoking and wood-burning stoves should also be eliminated. All of these measures require energy, time, and expenses for the family and child. The willingness of the child to comply with these adjustments will vary depending on the child's maturity and skills at finding acceptable substitute activities, and the parents' willingness and ability to perform these activities. Often environmental modifications will not provide immediate symptom improvement. This may also contribute to families' perception that environmental modifications were not helpful and promote poor adherence to the recommendation.

School Issues

The consequences of asthma on educational experiences often result in increased school absences due to illness episodes, repeated health care provider visits, and difficulties in illness management in the school setting. School absences have been used as a crude index of asthma morbidity, that is, an indication of children's response to treatment or undertreatment of the condition (Doull, Williams, Freezer, & Holgate, 1996), as well as a variable to describe the developmental and socialization impacts of the chronic condition. School absences interfere not only with educational experiences during childhood, but are also seen to have a profound impact on the framework for critical skill development in the adult years in career, employment, family, and overall life satisfaction.

Children with asthma miss twice as many days as other children on average. Illness-related absences have increased from 5.6 days in 1979–1981 to more than 11 days in 1990 (Taylor & Newacheck, 1992). Regardless of gender or ethnicity, children with asthma have more school absences than children without asthma. Asthma-related absences, however, are most common in the younger school-age children and decrease with age. School absences due to chronic illness are higher in female (Fowler, Johnson, & Atkinson, 1985) and African American children (Weiss, Gergen, & Hodfson, 1992; Gergen, Mullally, & Evans, 1988).

School absences have a major impact on parents' daily lives, both in terms of employment time and parental caregiving responsibilities. Parental unemployment, as evidenced by loss of workdays by parents, represents the largest single indirect cost of asthma (Weiss, Sullivan, & Lyttle, 2000). Parental burdens of childhood asthma include $4.64 billion in lost caregiver wages attributable to asthma-related school absences. In addition, children with asthma require close health care surveillance, necessitating multiple contacts with health care providers, thus children with asthma experience an increased number of school absences for clinic visits. For many families, daily home treatments and health care visits typically rests with the mothers (Turner-Henson, Holaday, & Swan, 1992).

Management of asthma while the child is at school often includes several problem areas. These may include school personnel's lack of knowledge of asthma and its management, difficulty in teacher-parent communication about asthma care, and under- and overrestrictiveness of students with asthma during physical education.

Children with asthma have been shown to have a moderately increased risk for learning disabilities. Children from lower income families have twice the risk for grade failure (Fowler, Davenport, & Garg, 1992). Children with asthma, as well as other children with chronic illness-related absences are likely to earn lower grades (O'Neil, Barysh, & Setear, 1985). Cadman and associates (1987) found more school-based problems in chronically ill children with disability than in those without.

In addition, strategies are needed to educate children, parents and educators in effective management and coping skills for the student with asthma. Programs such as the American Lung Association's Open Airways (www. lungusa.org) is a school-based curriculum that focuses on asthma education for the child with asthma, school peers and school personnel. School-based programs are needed to improve parent-teacher communication about care of asthmatic children, increase school personnel's knowledge about asthma management, and provide strategies to adapt school programs such as physical education programs to accommodate children with asthma. Warm-up periods (6–10 min) prior to exercise, as well as monitoring symptoms during exercise are recommended for children with asthma (U.S. Department of Health and Human Services [DHHS], 2001). Some children with asthma need medication prior to exercise. Programs that emphasize self-management skills have been shown to decrease absences (Perrin, MacLean, & Perrin, 1989; Perrin, Ma-cLean, Gortmaker, et al., 1992). In other short-term school-based interventions, the involvement of school nurses and peak flow monitoring did not significantly decrease school absences. However, it did reduce children's anxiety with asthma management in the school setting (Persaud et al., 1996). Stress management positively affected psychological outcomes and other aspects of functioning, but not school absences (Perrin, MacLean, Gortmaker, et al., 1992).

PARENT FACTORS

As a chronic condition, asthma requires daily monitoring, self-care management, and modifications in children's and families' daily lives. Coupled with the usual demands of family life (e.g., individual family member personnel care needs, school work, recreational activities, etc.), the addition of asthma caregiving demands make parenting even more difficult and challenging. For these parents, asthma caregiving responsibilities are added to normal and routine parenting responsibilities (Turner-Henson, Holaday, & Swan, 1992). Although the literature is inconclusive and presents contradictory findings, psychologic distress in parents, strained marital relationships, maternal depression, and distress in families with a chronically ill child have been reported. There is strong evidence that much of the distress results from the daily, practical demands of parenting a child with chronic conditions, such as asthma, and that it is more pronounced in women than in men (Holaday & Turner-Henson, 1991).

Self-efficacy or the confidence to perform recommended asthma management measures has been shown to be a strong predictor of various health outcomes (Wilson, Mitchell, & Rolnick, 1993). In the case of pediatric asthma, parents need to have the confidence to perform the daily asthma management therapies. Wilson, Mitchell, and Rolnick (1993) found that parents of young children with asthma often held a number of beliefs that interfered with asthma management. These beliefs included: periodic crises are to be expected and require emergency department services, medicines are not efficacious, asthma is an acute (not chronic) condition, and asthma is not serious. Parental caregiving of children with asthma requires that parents understand that asthma is a disease in which there is airway inflammation and that there is a need for daily monitoring and treatment, even in the absence of daily symptoms. Inaccurate beliefs about asthma are more likely to be seen in parents of children with mild asthma in which there are no daily symptoms or daily need for quick relief medications. Adherence to prescribed therapies, such as watching for asthma symptoms, managing symptoms (e.g., inhaler use prior to exercise), or making environmental modifications in the absence of daily asthma symptoms, is often difficult for families.

Caregiving in pediatric asthma is generally the responsibility of the child's mother, who maintains primary responsibility for the daily medical treatments and illness management, in addition to fulfilling the usual demands of household and employer expectations (Holaday & Turner-Henson, 1991). With the growing number of single-parent families, where the mother is usually the head of the household and primary income source, parenting demands are even further complicated.

Deficiencies in asthma management behaviors have been documented and are thought to play a significant role in pediatric asthma morbidity and mortality (Wilson, Mitchell, & Rolnick, 1993). Long-term medication regimens are difficult and costly (monthly medication costs average between $60–$120), and in asthma, where these regimens require daily medications and changes in lifestyle behaviors (e.g., smoking cessation, removal of family pets, etc.), adherence issues are even more complex. Parental attitudes such as apathy, failure to obtain necessary medications and supplies, anger related to the social stigma of having a child with asthma, and others can lead to increased asthma morbidity for children and adolescents. Cultural values and norms will also impact the family (and the parental caregiver) and expectations for health behaviors (Asch-Goodkin, 2000).

While nonadherence to management therapies even in the mild diagnostic categories can result in increased asthma morbidity, adherence to prescribed management therapies in the absence of daily reminders that "my child really does have asthma" may be the most difficult behavioral action for parents (Sherman & Hendeles, 1999). The intermittent nature of pediatric asthma has many implications for management adherence, particularly in the areas of medications and environmental modifications (Renne & Creer, 1985). In mild intermittent asthma there may be long periods of time between acute exacerbations (i.e., asthma attacks) and children/parents may forget the instructions for medication use, not carry the needed supplies or be unprepared for such occasions. Also, intermittent asthma episodes may generate different expectations on the part of the child and parent, thus they may fail to recognize the seriousness of the asthma episode that could potentially result in greater morbidity. In these situations the absence of daily asthma symptoms does not provide the behavioral stimuli to promote adherence.

Parental decision making is another important component to consider in pediatric asthma care. Daily decision making, such as symptom prevention, medication adjustments, crisis management, and use of medical and educational resources, are all important factors for the parent to consider. The decision-making process continues through a child's life, though as the child grows older, the responsibility for decision making needs to be transferred to the child.

ENVIRONMENTAL FACTORS

Children have physical and developmental characteristics that place them at greater risk for exposure to certain types of environmental agents. Epidemiological data have clearly documented an increase in severity of pediatric asthma and exposure to environmental variables such as allergens (e.g., dust mites, cockroach, pet allergen, molds, etc.), air pollution, and passive smoke (Bates, 1995). While research on environmental factors and pediatric asthma has primarily focused on home setting and environmental irritants, such as allergens (e.g., cockroach, dust mite, pet allergens, molds) and passive smoke, researchers are now beginning to examine the impact of environmental irritants in other settings, such as school environments.

Environmental allergen exposure in home settings has been clearly documented to contribute to asthma exacerbations in children. Children residing in areas that are crowded urban, older homes, or areas where the homes are old and often poorly maintained, are at greater risk for increased allergen exposure leading to increased asthma morbidity. A greater risk for environmental allergens and hazards has been documented in low-income environments, and families in these environments often have less control over their own physical surroundings (e.g., home maintenance) (Mott, 1995).

Children and adolescents spend a large percentage of their time in school settings, thus the school setting is the child's occupational setting. Clinical strategies and public policy are beginning to address the impact of school settings on children's health and particularly children with asthma. As previously noted, allergens and air pollution can impact pediatric asthma, though few studies have examined these environmental variables in school settings. vanWijnen and colleagues (1997) found cockroach at detectable levels in school dust samples; however, cockroach threshold levels capable of inducing sensitization or asthma exacerbation has not been defined. School-age children may have relatively high ambient pollution exposures, in part because they are physically active outdoors at the times when afternoon air pollution levels (e.g., ozone) are at their highest (Bates, 1995). Ozone at very low levels provokes airway inflammation, and as particulate air pollution increases there is an associated reduction in lung function. Linn and associates (1996) found that children experienced slight lung function changes in association with day-to-day air quality changes. While the short-term effects of air pollution appear to be small, the long-term effects are still unknown with respect to children who have asthma.

Increasing pediatric asthma morbidity, particularly among inner city and minority populations, has lead to interventions that focus on the school setting. As discussed earlier, the American Lung Association's Open Airways program focuses on asthma education in the school setting. The Environmental Protection Agency, in cooperation with multiple agencies (American Federation of Teachers, Association of School Business Officials, Council for American Private Education, National Education Association, National Parent Teachers Association, and the American Lung Association), has instituted the program, Indoor Air Quality (IAQ) Tools for Schools (available at: http:// www.epa.gov/iaq/schools/index.html). The IAQ Tools for Schools assists school personnel in carrying out a practical plan of action to prevent and resolve indoor air problems at little or no cost, using straightforward activities and school personnel. Key to this program is the involvement of all members of the school team, including the administrative staff (e.g., principal), teachers, parents, and custodial staff in examining the school environment. While the influence of school environments on pediatric asthma still remains unknown, this program seeks to improve indoor air quality in school settings through a coordinated school effort focusing on both prevention and action activities.

Smoking and Pediatric Asthma

Passive smoke exposure is a highly prevalent respiratory irritant, and its impact in children's health, particularly increased asthma morbidity, has been clearly documented (Gergen, Fowler, Maurer, Davis, & Overpeck, 1998). A significant number of children are exposed to passive smoke exposure, ranging from 24% during pregnancy (maternal smoking) to 43% of young children (ages 2 months–11 years) who live in a household with at least one smoker (Pirkle et al., 1996). Younger children experience the greatest risk from passive smoke exposure as evidenced by increased morbidity and increased health care costs. Increased rates of medical services and hospitalizations are seen in young children who are exposed to passive smoke, particularly those children with asthma (Stoddard & Gray, 1997). Recovery from acute asthma exacerbations in children can be impaired significantly by passive smoke exposure, and ongoing exposure in children is characterized by persistent asthma symptoms (Abulhosh, Morray, Llewellyn, & Redding, 1997).

Maternal smoking can have the strongest impact on children's overall health (Henschen et al., 1997; Stoddard & Gray, 1997). Annual direct medical expenditures for childhood respiratory illness attributable to maternal smoking has been estimated to total $661 million for children under the age of 6 years (Stoddard & Gray, 1997). Coupled with the impact of pediatric asthma on family budgets (reduced parental productivity from increased number of children's sick days), family out-of-pocket expenditures (e.g., costs for travel, extra meals, babysitters, etc.) result in the largest single indirect cost of childhood asthma (Taggart & Fullwood, 1993; Weiss, Sullivan, & Lyttle, 2000).

Smoking Cessation and Pediatric Settings

The National Asthma Education and Prevention Program Expert Panel report (NHLBI, 1997) listed cigarette smoking as the most common and preventable environmental trigger for asthma exacerbation. Despite the expert panel's strong recommendations, passive smoke exposure in pediatric asthma remains a major problem. These recommendations provide direction for clinical intervention, focusing primarily on educational interventions. Education programs alone may impact parental smoking behaviors, though the success and sustained abstinence rates are variable (Winkelstein, Tarzian, & Wood, 1997; Donnelly, Donnelly, & Thong, 1987). Others have noted that educational smoking cessation programs may not have a significant impact on smoking cessation success, in that parents who do not perceive smoking as impacting the child's asthma are less likely to attend (Fish, Wilson, Latini, & Starr, 1996). Smoking cessation programs that use minimal contact and those using feedback (e.g., child's urine cotinine) strategies have had limited success, and quit rates are still low (McIntosh, Clark, & Howatt, 1994). Other programs have sought to examine parental environmental modifications to reduce passive smoke exposure in the home (e.g., smoking outside, smoking only when child is not home, etc.) (Winkelstein, Tarzian, & Wood, 1997). However, significant reductions in children's urine cotinine levels were not found, nor were there significant reductions in parental smoking. Behavioral intervention for parents who smoke have reported greater reductions in passive smoke exposure (Wahlgren, Hovell, Meltzer, Hofstetter, & Zakarian, 1997), though these interventions need to address other potential sources of passive smoke (such as other household members or visitors who may smoke).

Role of Providers in Smoking Cessation Interventions

Much of the research in smoking cessation in pediatric settings has focused on the role of the physician as counselor. The American Academy of Pediatrics (1997) published a position paper profiling the harmful impact of passive smoke on children and urging pediatricians to incorporate passive smoke exposure assessments and counseling into their clinical practices. Primary care settings and well child care provide opportunities for health professionals to intervene with parents in smoking cessation.

Few pediatric settings have consistently addressed smoking cessation counseling for parents of children with asthma. Smoking cessation counseling by health professionals (e.g., pediatricians, pediatric nurses) remains a major problem. Frankowski, Weaver, and Secker-Walker (1993) identified four barriers reported by pediatricians in smoking cessation counseling: failure to identify parents, perception that parents would react negatively, lack of time, and lack of training. Health professionals in pediatric settings often lack the skills to provide smoking cessation counseling (Klein, Portilla, Goldstein, & Leininger, 1995; Turner-Henson et al., 1999). However, training on effective behavior change concepts and enhancing self-efficacy to deliver counseling messages should be the major focus rather than an educational message.

Smoking cessation strategies have been implemented primarily focused in adult settings. Studies using nurses or health educators to supplement physician advice have been promising, however, these studies have focused primarily on adult settings with few reports of programs in pediatric settings. Clinical practice strategies that include assessment of parental smoking status, that is, smoking status of household members inquired about at each clinical encounter (also referred to as smoking as a vital sign) (Turner-Henson et al., 1999), and interventions that target the sources of children's passive smoke exposure are greatly need in pediatric settings.

HEALTH PROMOTION AND DISABILITY PREVENTION IN PEDIATRIC ASTHMA

Health promotion and disability prevention in children and adolescents with asthma, such as decreasing sedentary lifestyles and improving physical fitness, are of great concern for health care professionals. Physical fitness programs for asthmatic children have been successful in improving physical fitness parameters and vital capacity (Orenstein, Reed, Grogan, & Crawford, 1985), while decreasing school absences and improving sociability, self-assertion, and peer acceptance (Szentagothai, Gyene, Szocaska, & Osvath, 1987). Severely asthmatic children with decreased physical fitness levels can achieve normal cardiopulmonary fitness and increase work tolerance after training (Ludwick, Jones, Jones, Fukuhara, & Strunk, 1986). Fitness training programs have not been shown to change the severity of the disease or pulmonary functions studies (Goldberg, 1990; Varray & Prefault, 1992).

While a positive attitude toward physical activity in children and adolescents with asthma may be associated with greater active involvement, many other factors may contribute to decreased physical activity in children and adolescents with asthma. Children and adolescents with asthma are often excluded from physical activity, in both organized sports and vigorous free play (Newacheck & Halfon, 1998). This exclusion may be due to parents, physicians, physical education teachers, or even their own reluctance to provoke an attack of *exercise-induced asthma* (EIA is narrowing of the airway which occurs after the onset of vigorous activity, due to airway hyper reactivity present in asthma).

For children and adolescents with asthma, EIA may be prevented with premedicating prior to exercise with inhaled $beta_2$-agonist (e.g., Albuterol) and/or cromolyn before preexercise and additional $beta_2$-agonist inhalation for symptom relief as needed. EIA occurs in about 85% of individuals with asthma who have limited airflow and in about 73% of those with asthma who have normal lung function before exercise. Approximately half of individuals with asthma who are well controlled with normal lung function require prophylactic therapy for EIA, and another third may require intermittent treatment after exercise. Parental reports of EIA, even among known children and adolescents with asthma, have been found to be poor predictors of the presence or absence of EIA (Branford, McNutt, & Fink, 1991); therefore, the existence of EIA may not be a predictor of physical activity in children and adolescents with asthma.

Researchers have demonstrated that activity patterns and fitness are influenced not only by social and environmental factors but also by a variety of personal attributes. Physical activity has long been considered beneficial to children's psychomotor development (Malina, 1990), socialization (Sage, 1991), cognitive development, self-esteem (Weiss, McAuley, & Ebbeck, 1990), and general well-being (Simons-Morton, Parcel, & O'Hara, 1988). In the case of physical activity, the involvement of children appears to be related to parental encouragement of participation (Holaday & Turner-Henson, 1991). Support from the family, peers, friends, teachers, and coaches also seem to prompt participation. Patterns of participation in physical activity also vary by gender and race (Holaday & Turner-Henson, 1991). Most of the research on the beneficial effects of physical activity, however, has been done with the healthy school age population or with young athletes. There is less information on the potential benefits of enhanced physical activity and fitness for the children and adolescents with asthma.

The Impact of a Sedentary Lifestyle in Pediatric Asthma

Researchers have clearly demonstrated that chronic disease morbidity and mortality linked to sedentary lifestyles in adults is predictable and costly, though the relationships for children and adolescents with asthma have not been carefully explored. National surveys have shown, that in combination with dietary patterns, physical inactivity ranks along with tobacco use among the leading preventable contributors of mortality for Americans (McGinnis, 1992). Studies conducted in the past two decades have convincingly demonstrated a link between the level of daily, physical activity in adults and decreased incidence of cardiovascular morbidity and mortality (Blair et al., 1993).

Among adults physical inactivity has been identified as one of the most important modifiable risk factors related to morbidity and mortality. Increased levels of physical fitness and activity have also been found to decrease risks for cardiovascular morbidity and mortality in chronically ill adults (Barlow, Kohl, & Blair, 1993). The benefits of exercise for adults have been linked to improved functional capacity and cardiovascular efficiency, a reduction in physiologic and metabolic atherogenic risk factors, and an improved psychological well-being (Haskell et al., 1992). The anticipated national benefits from greater physical activity and fitness include reductions in both direct (hospital care, service of physicians and nurses, drugs, public health services, insurance costs) and indirect costs (loss of production from illness, premature death), and an improvement in overall lifestyle (Shephard, 1990).

Aerobic fitness in children has steadily declined by 10% over the past decade (Updyke & Willett, 1989), and an increasing incidence in obesity has been noted (Gortmaker, Dietz, & Cheung, 1990). Coupled with lifestyle behaviors, environmental factors, such as inner city life, have been noted to influence physical fitness as evidenced by decreased levels of cardiovascular endurance (Zhu & Krause, 1993). Researchers have found that children with chronic conditions have increased morbidity during childhood that has been associated with poor health rating in adulthood (ratio 1:38) (Power & Peckham, 1990). The relationships between health ratings in childhood and adulthood are not known for children with asthma. However, based on what is known for healthy individuals, the health risks for children and adolescents with asthma, especially those associated with sedentary lifestyles and chronic diseases, appear to track into adulthood, and the adult risks rooted in childhood could be potentially enhanced by sedentary lifestyles.

The establishment of a regular program of physical activities could improve muscular strength, muscular endurance, flexibility and cardiorespiratory fitness in children and youth with asthma. This could in turn improve abilities to perform tasks of daily living, reduce the total burden of ill health during school-age and adolescent years, encourage the development of a physically active lifestyle, and reduce future morbidity costs. Recommendations for physical activity and children with asthma can be found in the *Bright Futures in Practice: Physical Activity* publication (www.brightfutures.org).

SUMMARY

Asthma morbidity in children and adolescents is rapidly increasing despite major improvements in treatment and control. The public health burden of pediatric asthma is growing and health care costs, as well as costs to the developing child are alarming. The development of strategies in pediatric asthma care must take into consideration "the existence and unrealized potential of ecologies that sustain and strengthen constructive processes in society, the family, and the self" (Bronfenbrenner, 1986, p. 738). In order to create environments that are conducive to healthy care and parenting behaviors in pediatric asthma, it is proposed that health professionals address the specific areas:

- symptom management demands on children and adolescents, taking into account the motor skills required (e.g., inhalers with spacers) and decision making skills required in emergency situations;
- influences of daily life activities of children and adolescents, specifically the impact on school functioning, focusing on the need to reduce school absences;
- heavy time burdens and demands on family caregivers, particularly the burdens for mothers as primary caregivers;

- time constraints and resources on families, particularly in single-parent families and employed mothers;
- development of interventions to promote adherence in symptom management focusing on behavioral strategies which incorporate both the child with asthma and parent behaviors (medication administration, environmental triggers such as smoking, and so forth); and
- development of interventions that promote healthy physical environments, such as quality indoor air (home and school settings) for children and adolescents with asthma.

As recognized by the National Asthma Education and Prevention Program (NHLBI, 1997b), health care professionals can only address these areas through an established and ongoing partnership with the child and family in asthma care. These partnerships are essential in controlling and reducing the daily consequences of asthma on children's and families' lives. It is essential that the health care professional recognize the key role that both the child and family have in maintaining asthma control that promotes a healthy lifestyle.

REFERENCES

Abulhosh, R. S., Morray, B. H., Llewellyn, C. L., & Redding, G. J. (1997). Passive smoke exposure impairs recovery after hospitalization for acute asthma. *Archives of Pediatric and Adolescent Medicine, 15,* 135–139.

American Academy of Asthma, Allergy and Immunology. (1999). *Update on pediatric asthma: Promoting best practice.* Available at: http://www.aaaai.org/professional/initiatives/pediatricasthma.stm

American Academy of Pediatrics. (1997). Environmental tobacco smoke: A hazard to children. *Pediatrics, 99,* 639–642.

American Lung Association. (2001). Prevalence based on revised National Health Interview survey. Available at: http://www.lungusa.org/data/data_102000.html

Asch-Goodkin, J. (2000). Caring for diverse populations: Eliminating disparities in asthma management. *Patient Care Nurse Practitioner, 3,* 68–70, 72, 74.

Barlow, C. E., Kohl, H. W., & Blair, S. N. (1993). Physical fitness and cardiovascular disease mortality in men with chronic disease. *Journal of the American College of Sports Medicine, 25*(Suppl.), 75. Abstract.

Bates, D. V. (1995). Observations on asthma. *Environmental Health Perspectives, 103,* 243–247.

Blair, S. N., Kohl, H. W., & Barlow, C. E. (1993). Physical activity, physical fitness, and all-cause mortality in women: Do women need to be active? *Journal of the American College of Nutrition, 12,* 368–371.

Branford, R. P., McNutt, G. M., & Fink, J. N. (1991). Exercise-induced asthma in adolescent gym class population. *International Archives of Allergy and Applied Immunology, 94*, 272–274.

Bronfenbrenner, U. (1986). Ecology of the family as a context for human development. *Developmental Psychology, 22*, 723–742.

Brook, U., Stein, D., & Alkalay, Y. (1994). The attitude of asthmatic and nonasthmatic adolescents toward gymnastic lessons at school. *Journal of Asthma, 31*, 171–175.

Cadman, D., Boule, M., Szatmari, P., et al. (1987). Chronic illness, disability, and mental and social well-being. *Pediatrics, 79*, 805–813.

Centers for Disease Control. (1998). Asthma—United States, 1980–1990. *MMWR, Morbitity and Mortality Weekly Report, 41*, 733–735.

Cunningham, J., O'Connor, G. T., Dockery, D. W., & Speizer, F. E. (1996). Environmental tobacco smoke, wheezing, and asthma in children in 24 communities. *American Journal of Respiratory & Critical Care Medicine, 153*, 218–224.

Donnelly, J. E., Donnelly, W. J., & Thong, Y. H. (1987). Parental perceptions and attitudes toward asthma and its treatment: A controlled study. *Social Science & Medicine, 24*, 431–437.

Doull, I. J., Williams, A. A., Freezer, N. J., & Holgate, S. T. (1996). Descriptive study of cough, wheeze and school absence in childhood. *Thorax, 51*, 630–631.

Eggleston, P. A. (1998). Urban children and asthma: Morbidity and mortality. *Immunology & Allergy Clinics of North America, 18*, 75–84.

Fish, L., Wilson, S. R., Latini, D. M., & Starr, N. J. (1996). An education program for parents of children with asthma: Differences in attendance between smoking and nonsmoking parents. *American Journal of Public Health, 86*, 246–248.

Fowler, M. G., Davenport, M. G., & Garg, R. (1992). School functioning of U.S. children with asthma. *Pediatrics, 90*, 939–944.

Fowler, M., Johnson, M., & Atkinson, S. (1985). School achievement and absence in children with chronic health conditions. *Journal of Pediatrics, 106*, 683–687.

Frankowski, B. L., Weaver, S. O., & Secker-Walker, R. H. (1993). Advising parents to stop smoking: Pediatricians' and parents' attitudes. *Pediatrics, 91*, 296–300.

Gergen, P. J., Fowler, J. A., Maurer, K. R., Davis, W. W., & Overpeck, M. D. (1998). The burden of environmental tobacco smoke exposure on the respiratory health of children 2 months through 5 years of age in the United States: Third National Health and Nutrition Examination Survey, 1988 to 1994. *Pediatrics, 101*, e8.

Gergen, P., Mullally, D., & Evans, R. (1988). National survey of prevalence of asthma among children in the United States: 1976 to 1980. *Pediatrics, 81*, 1–7.

Goldberg, B. (1990). Children, sports, and chronic disease. *Physician Sportsmedicine, 18*, 44–56.

Gortmaker, S. L., Dietz, W. H., & Cheung, L. W. Y. (1990). Inactivity, diet, and the fattening of America. *Journal of the American Dietetic Association, 90*, 1247–1255.

Haskell, W. L., Leon, A. S., Caspersen, C. J., Froelicher, V. F., Hagberg, J. M., Harlan, W., Holloszy, J. O., Regensteiner, J. G., Thompson, P. D., Washburn, R. A., & Wilson, F. W. F. (1992). Cardiovascular benefits and assessment of physical activity and physical fitness in adults. *Medicine and Science in Sports and Exercise, 24*, 201–220.

Henschen, M., Frischer, T., Pracht, T., Spiekerkotter, E., Karmaus, W., Meinert, R., Lehnert, W., Wehrle, E., & Kuehr, J. (1997). The internal dose of passive smoking at home depends on the size of the dwelling. *Environmental Research, 72*, 65–71.

Holaday, B., & Turner-Henson, A. (1991). *Growing up and going out: A survey of chronically ill children's use of time out-of-school.* Final research report for MCI 060550 Maternal and Child Health Program (Title V, Social Security Act, Health Resources and Services Administration, Department of Health and Human Services).

Institute of Medicine Committee on the Assessment of Asthma and Indoor Air, Division of Health Promotion and Disease Prevention. (2000). *Clearing the air: Asthma and indoor air exposures.* Washington, DC: National Academy Press.

Klein, J. D., Portilla, M., Goldstein, A., & Leininger, L. (1995). Training pediatric residents to prevent tobacco use. *Pediatrics, 96*, 326–330.

Landau, L. I. (1996). Risks of developing asthma. *Pediatric Pulmonology, 22*, 314–418.

LeSouef, P. (1997). Genetics of asthma: What do we need to know? *Pediatric Pulmonology, 15*, 3–8.

Linn, W. S., Shamoo, D. A., Anderson, K. R., Peng, R. C., Avol, E. L., Hackeny, J. D., & Gong, H. Jr. (1996). Short-term air pollution exposures and responses in Los Angeles schoolchildren. *Journal of Exposure Analyses & Environmental Epidemiology, 6*, 449–472.

Lozano, P., Connell, F. A., & Koepsell, T. D. (1995). Use of health services by African-American children with asthma on Medicaid. *Journal of the American Medical Association, 274*, 469–473.

Lozano, P., Sullivan, S. D., Smith, D. H., & Weiss, K. B. (1999). The economic burden of asthma in U.S. children: Estimates from the National Medical Expenditure survey. *Journal of Allergy & Clinical Immunology, 104,* 957–963.

Ludwick, S. K., Jones, J. W., Jones, T. K., Fukuhara, J. T., & Strunk, R. C. (1986). Normalization of cardiopulmonary endurance in severely asthmatic children after bicycle ergometry therapy. *Journal of Pediatrics, 109*, 446–451.

Malina, R. M. (1990). Growth, exercise, fitness and later outcomes. In C. Bouchard, R. J. Shephard, & T. Stephens (Eds.), *Exercise, fitness and health* (pp. 637–653). Champaign, IL: Human Genetics.

McGinnis, J. M. (1992). The public health burden of a sedentary life style. *Medicine & Science in Sports and Exercise, 24*(6 Suppl.), 196–200.

McIntosh, N. A., Clark, N. M., & Howatt, W. F. (1994). Reducing tobacco smoke in the environment of the child with asthma: A cotinine-assisted, minimal-contact intervention. *Journal of Asthma, 31*, 453–462.

Mott, L. (1995). The disproportionate impact of environmental health threats on children of color. *Environmental Health Perspectives, 103*, 33–35.

Murray, M. D., Stang, P., & Tierney, W. M. (1997). Health care use by inner-city patients with asthma. *Journal of Clinical Epidemiology, 50*, 167–174.

National Center for Health Statistics. (1986). Advance data from vital and health statistics: National Ambulatory Medical Care Survey, DHHS Publication No. PHS 87–2350, Washington, DC: U.S. Government Printing Office.

National Heart, Lung and Blood Institute. (1997a). *Practical guide for the diagnosis and management of asthma.* (NIH Publication No. 97–4053). Washington, DC: U.S. Government Printing Office.

National Heart, Lung and Blood Institute. (1997b). *Guidelines for the diagnosis and management of asthma. National Asthma Education Program Expert Panel Report II.* (NIH Publication No. 97-4051A). Washington, DC: U.S. Government Printing Office.

Newacheck, P. W., Budetti, P. P., & Halfon, N. (1986). Trends in activity limiting chronic conditions among children. *American Journal of Public Health, 76,* 178–184.

Newacheck, P. W., & Halfon, N. (1998). Prevalence and impact of disabling chronic conditions in childhood. *American Journal of Public Health, 88,* 610–617.

O'Neil, S., Barysh, N., & Setear S. (1985). Determining school programming needs of special population groups: A study of asthmatic children. *Journal of School Health, 55,* 237–239.

Orenstein, D. M., Reed, M. E., Grogan, F. T., Jr., & Crawford, L. V. (1985). Exercise conditioning in children with asthma. *Journal of Pediatrics, 106,* 556–560.

Perrin, J. M., MacLean, W. E., Jr., Gortmaker, S. L., Asher, K. N., et al. (1992). Improving the psychological status of children with asthma: A randomized controlled trial. *Developmental and Behavioral Pediatrics, 13,* 241–247.

Perrin, J. M., MacLean, W. E., Jr., & Perrin, E. C. (1989). Parental perceptions of health status and psychologic adjustment of children with asthma. *Pediatrics, 83,* 26–30.

Persaud, D. I., Barnett, S. E., Weller, S. C., Baldwin, C. D., Niebuhr, V., & McCormick, D. P. (1996). An asthma self-management program for children, including instruction in peak flow monitoring by school nurses. *Journal of Asthma, 33,* 37–43.

Pirkle, J. L., Flegal, K. M., Bernert, J. T., Brody, D. J., Etzel, R. A., & Maurer, K. R. (1996). Exposure of the U.S. population to environmental tobacco smoke: The third National Health and Nutrition Examination Survey, 1988 to 1991. *Journal of the American Medical Association, 275,* 1233–1240.

Power, C., & Peckham, C. (1990). Childhood morbidity and adulthood ill health. *Journal of Epidemiology and Community Health, 44,* 69–74.

Renne, C. M., & Creer, T. L. (1985). Asthmatic children and their families. In M. L. Walraich & D. K. Routh (Eds.), *Advances in developmental and behavioral pediatrics* (pp. 41–81). Greenwich, CT: JAI Press.

Sage, G. H. (1991). A commentary on qualitative research as a form of scientific inquiry in sport and physical education. *Research Quarterly in Exercise and Sport, 60*(1), 25–29.

Shepard, R. J. (1990). Physical activity and cancer. *International Journal of Sports Medicine, 11,* 413–420.

Sherman, J. M., & Hendeles, L. (1999). Improving adherence to asthma medications. *Contemporary Pediatrics, 16,* 51–64.

Simons-Morton, B., Parcel, G., & O'Hara, N. (1988). Health-related physical fitness in childhood: Status and recommendations. *Annual Review of Public Health, 9,* 403–425.

Stoddard, J. J., & Gray, B. (1997). Maternal smoking and medical expenditure for childhood respiratory illness. *American Journal of Public Health, 87,* 205–209.

Szentagothai, K., Gyene, I., Szocska, M., & Osvath, P. (1987). Physical exercise program for children with bronchial asthma. *Pediatric Pulmonology, 3,* 166–172.

Taggart, V. S., & Fulwood, R. (1993). Youth health report card: Asthma. *Preventive Medicine, 22,* 579–584.

Taylor, W. R., & Newacheck, P. W. (1992). Impact of childhood asthma on health. *Pediatrics, 90,* 657–662.

Turner-Henson, A., Holaday, B., & Swan, J. (1992). When parenting becomes caregiving: Caring for the chronically ill child. *Family and Community Health, 15*, 19–30.

Turner-Henson, A., Kohler, C., O'Brien, J., Rodgers, T., Johnston, J., & Lyrene, R. (1998). Pediatric nurses' perceptions of smoking cessation counseling. *American Public Health Association Annual Meeting Proceedings* Abstract.

Turner-Henson, A., Kohler, C., Lyrene, R., O'Brien, J., Johnston, J., & Rodgers, T. F. (1999). Smoking status as a vital sign in pediatric settings (letter to editor). *Pediatrics, 103*, 1079–1080.

U.S. Department of Health and Human Services. (2001). *Bright futures in practice: Physical activity.* Washington, DC: National Center for Education in Maternal and Child Health, Georgetown University.

Updyke, W., & Willett, M. (1989). Physical fitness trends in American youth 1989–1990 [Press Release]. Bloomington, IN: Chrysler-AAU Physical Fitness Program.

vanWijnen, J. H., Verhoeff, A. P., Mulder-Folkerts, D. K., Brachel, H. J., & Schou, C. (1997). Cockroach allergen in house dust. *Allergy, 52*, 460–464.

Varray, A., & Prefaut, C. (1992). Importance of physical exercise training ion asthmatics. *Journal of Asthma, 29*, 229–234.

Wahlgren, D. R., Hovell, M. F., Meltzer, S. B., Hofstetter, C. R., & Zakarian, J. M. (1997). Reduction of environmental tobacco smoke exposure in asthmatic children: A 2-year follow-up. *Chest, 111*, 81–88.

Weiss, K., & Budetti, P. (1993). Examining issues in health care delivery for asthma: Background and workshop overview. *Medical Care, 31*, 9–19.

Weiss, K., Gergen, P., & Hodfson, T. (1992). An economic evaluation of asthma in the United States. *New England Journal of Medicine, 326*, 862–866.

Weiss, K. B., Sullivan, S. D., & Lyttle, C. S. (2000). Trends in the cost of illness for asthma in the United State, 1985–1994. *Journal of Allergy & Clinical Immunology, 106*, 493–499.

Weiss, M., McAuley, E., & Ebbeck, V. (1990). Self-esteem and causal attributions for children's physical and social competence in sport. *Journal of Sport and Exercise Psychology, 12*, 21–36.

Wilson, S. R., Mitchell, J. H., & Rolnick, S. (1993). Effective and ineffective management behaviors of parents of infants and young children with asthma. *Journal of Pediatric Psychology, 18*, 61–81.

Winkelstein, M. L., Tarzian, A., & Wood, R. A. (1997). Parental smoking behavior and passive smoke exposure in children with asthma. *Annals of Allergy, Asthma and Immunology, 78*, 419–423.

Zhu, W., & Krause, J. (1993). Physical fitness screening of inner-city children and youth. *Medicine and Science in Sports and Exercise*, 124 Abstract.

CHAPTER 2

Type 1 Diabetes

Terri H. Lipman

D iabetes mellitus is an ancient disease first described in the Ebers Papyrus of Egypt in 1500 B.C. Later, Aretaeus of Cappadocia, who lived from 81–138 A.D., named the disease *diabetes* from the Greek word meaning to flow through a siphon. He described diabetes as a "melting down of the flesh and limbs into urine" (Waife, 1980).

Diabetes mellitus is a disorder of glucose metabolism. The destruction of pancreatic beta cells (the insulin-secreting cells) results in a deficiency of insulin. Type 1 diabetes, or insulin-dependent diabetes mellitus (IDDM) is the most common endocrine disease in children, affecting about 120,000 individuals 0–19 years of age in the United States (LaPorte, Matsushima, & Chang, 1995). Although the discovery of injectable insulin in 1921 by Banting and Best made diabetes a treatable disorder, diabetes is still a major cause of mortality, severe morbidity, and decreased quality of life (Diabetes Epidemiology Research International Mortality Study Group, 1991).

The goal of diabetes prevention has fostered many studies attempting to identify the risk factors of Type 1 diabetes throughout the world. There is substantial geographical variability in the incidence of Type 1 diabetes. A review of the diabetes epidemiology research demonstrated a > 350-fold variation in the incidence among 100 populations worldwide (Karvonen et al., 2000). This geographic variability appears greater than that seen for nearly any other major chronic disease. The risk of Type 1 diabetes associated with place of residence is greater than the well known biologic risk factors of family history of disease and/or the presence of diabetes susceptibility genes (LaPorte, Matsushima, & Chang, 1995). Therefore, the ability to measure precisely the variability in different populations through epidemiologic methods may provide an important key to elucidating the causes of Type 1 diabetes.

ETIOLOGY

Autoimmunity

In autoimmunity, self-antigens are no longer recognized as such, and a self-destructive process occurs directed by one's own immune system (Volpe, 1985). The discovery that Type 1 diabetes is an autoimmune disease (i.e., caused by autoimmune destruction) and, therefore, autoimmunity is an agent of the disease, was derived from a series of observations. First, it was found that mononuclear cell infiltrates are present around and inside islet cells at the time of diagnosis (Gepts, 1965). Then it was found that islet cell antibodies are detected in the majority of newly diagnosed patients with Type 1 diabetes (Lendrum, Walker, & Gamble, 1975). In addition, it has been demonstrated that immunosuppressive agents cause remission of diabetes in newly diagnosed patients (Bougneres et al., 1988).

Autoimmunity can be used to denote the demonstration of an autoantibody directed against a self-antigen, more correctly termed *autoimmune response*. Autoantibodies may be present in persons who have no demonstrable disease. Alternatively, autoimmunity may describe a disease caused by an autoimmune response, also called an *autoimmune disease* (Rose & Mackay, 1985). It has been shown that when an at risk population of first degree relatives of persons with Type 1 diabetes are followed prospectively, evidence of an autoimmune response (presence of islet cell antibodies) may be present up to 9 years prior to the onset of clinically evident diabetes (Bingley, Bonifacio, & Gale, 1993). Data also show that islet cell antibodies in nonaffected at risk subjects may spontaneously disappear (Spencer et al., 1984), although high antibody titers are highly predictive (Karjalainen, 1990).

Another antibody found in 40% of newly diagnosed patents with Type 1 diabetes is insulin autoantibody (Atkinson et al., 1986). In addition, some patients with diabetes demonstrate glutamic acid decarboxylase (GAD) antibodies (Kaufman et al., 1992). GAD autoantibodies may prove to be highly predictive of Type 1 diabetes. Therefore, it appears that there are predisposing, or initiating risk factors in the host or the environment and precipitating environmental risk factors, occurring at different times, that are crucial in the progression along the immunity continuum.

Genetics

It is generally agreed that genetic susceptibility is a necessary precursor to the development of Type 1 diabetes. Studies of monozygotic twins indicate a concordance rate for Type 1 diabetes of 30–50% (Norris, Dorman, Lewis, & LaPorte, 1987; Olmos et al., 1988). The average risk of developing Type 1 diabetes in first degree family members is 4–7% (Wagener et al., 1982; Tarn et al., 1988). In comparison, the probability of developing Type 1 diabetes is 0.2% in the general population of the United States (Laporte et al., 1995). Therefore, the diabetogenic gene(s) seems to increase the risk of developing Type 1 diabetes by a factor of at least 20.

Studies of genetic markers called *human leukocyte antigens* have done much to elucidate the role of genes in the development of Type 1 diabetes. All tissue cells, with the exception of mature red blood cells, are genetically marked with a combination of histocompatibility antigens on the membrane surface. Because the white blood cells are examined for the identification of these antigens, they are also called human leukocyte antigens (HLA). Human leukocyte antigens are coded by genes called the major histocompatibility complex (MHC), located on chromosome number 6. These MHC genes are labeled A, B, C, and D. Class-1 molecules comprise the HLA type D and are produced only by macrophages and B lymphocytes. HLA class-2 antigens are on the surface of the macrophage close to the foreign antigen. This combination of foreign and class-2 antigens is needed for recognition of the helper T cells and causes activation of helper T cells. HLA class-1 antigens on the surface of infected cells are necessary for recognition and destruction by cytotoxic T cells. Endocrine autoimmunity is most closely associated with HLA class-2 antigens (HLA D and subgroup DR) (Fox, 1987).

It is believed that certain HLA genes play a role in genetic susceptibility, rather than cause inheritance of autoimmunity. There is a well documented association between HLA-DR and autoimmunity in humans. It is unknown whether HLA antigens themselves predispose to autoimmunity or whether there are yet undefined autoimmunogenic genes located close to, and inherited with, the DR locus genes (Raffel & Rotter, 1985). Individuals with Type 1 diabetes have an increased frequency of HLA genes B 8, B 15, DR3, and DR4. Ninety-five percent of whites with Type 1 diabetes have DR3 and/or DR4 (Eisenbarth, 1986). However, the likelihood that an individual in the general population who has DR3 or DR4 will develop Type 1 diabetes is 2.5% that of a person with DR3 or DR4 and a first degree relative with Type 1 diabetes (Faas & Trucco, 1994a, 1994b).

Knowledge of HLA antigens is extremely important for the study of the inheritance of Type 1 diabetes. If one child in a family has Type 1 diabetes, the risk of diabetes in the siblings is related to the number of HLA haplotypes the sibling shares with the diabetic child. If the children are HLA identical (i.e., two haplotypes are shared with the diabetic sibling) the risk of developing diabetes is approximately 16–25%; if one haplotype is shared it is 5–7%; and if neither haplotype is shared it is 1–2%, which is still 10 times > 0.2% risk in the general population (Scheuner, Raffel, & Rotter, 1997). Factors other than genetics must influence the transmission of susceptibility to Type 1 diabetes. Although monozygotic twins of children with Type 1 diabetes are genetically identical to the diabetic child, at least 50% do not develop diabetes.

Studies at the DNA level have added much information on the genetic transmission of Type 1 diabetes. It has been shown that the HLA-DQ locus contains some of the strongest known risk markers and protective alleles (Thorsby & Ronningen, 1993). Morel and colleagues (1988) demonstrated that individuals who do not have an aspartic acid in position 57 (Asp-57) of their HLA-DQ beta chain have a relative risk of 10% or less of developing Type 1 diabetes. The 20-fold increased incidence of Type 1 diabetes in Allegheny County compared to China appears to be related to the high prevalence of the non-Asp-57 marker in the Chinese (Bao, Wang, Dorman, & Trucco, 1989). Although this does not fully explain the inheritance of Type 1 diabetes, it is more sensitive than HLA typing in assessing the risk of Type 1 diabetes.

ENVIRONMENTAL FACTORS

Dietary Factors

Nitrosamines

Helgason and Jonassen (1981) noted a much higher than expected incidence of Type 1 diabetes in Icelandic boys born in October. The authors proposed that there was an environmental agent, which affected the mother at the time of conception or early in fetal life when the fetal pancreas is most susceptible to injury. They postulated that the large amount of smoked mutton containing the food additive N-nitroso that is consumed in Iceland at Christmas time produced diabetes in those progeny conceived at that time. They proposed that N-nitroso was a diabetogenic agent, affecting parental germ cells. This hypothesis was supported by a study in which N-nitroso was given to mice during conception and diabetes occurred in the progeny (Helgason, Ewen, Ross, & Stowers, 1982).

Infant Feeding

A study from Norway and Sweden has shown that a smaller proportion of children with Type 1 diabetes have ever been breast-fed, and that children with Type 1 diabetes were breast-fed shorter periods of time compared to their healthy siblings (Borch-Johnson et al., 1984). An inverse correlation was demonstrated between breast-feeding nadir and Type 1 diabetes incidence in childhood. The time lag between the breast-feeding nadir and Type 1 diabetes incidence peak in Norway was approximately 9 years—close to the average age of onset of Type 1 diabetes in that population. There is accumulating evidence that early introduction to Northern European cow's milk protein may be an important factor in inducing the expression of diabetes in genetically predisposed infants (Gerstein, 1994). Early ingestion of bovine serum albumin may induce beta cell inflammatory responses (Karjalainen et al., 1992).

Exposure to Infectious Agents

The primary infectious agent postulated to be associated with diabetes is a virus. The possible role of a virus in the etiology of Type 1 diabetes was first suggested in 1899 (Craighead, 1978). In the 1920s an increased incidence of diabetes was noted in Scandinavia after outbreaks of mumps virus infection (Gundersen, 1927). Other studies have shown similar increases (Sultz, Hart, & Zielenzny, 1975), but a drastic reduction in the incidence of mumps since the initiation of the mumps vaccine has not resulted in a major decrease in the incidence of diabetes (Bennett, 1985). There is a question of whether the vaccine itself may be an antecedent to diabetes. A study in Finland (after MMR vaccination) showed an increase of Type 1 diabetes (after MMR vaccination) (Hyoty et al., 1993).

Proponents of the theory that a virus causes diabetes or precipitates the autoimmune response believe that this factor helps to explain the seasonality of Type 1 diabetes. The onset of diabetes peaks in the midwinter and has a nadir in the spring. This characteristic is observed in both northern and southern hemispheres and in high and low risk populations. Type 1 diabetes has greater prevalence in cold climates where viral infections are more common. In addition, viral infections in children are most common in the early school-aged years and during adolescence, which are also the peak years for the onset of Type 1 diabetes (Fohlman & Friman, 1993). This may be associated with early infection with a slow virus. A viral etiology could also explain epidemics of Type 1 diabetes. Evidence of recent infection by the coxsackie B virus was demonstrated in a number of Swedish children with new onset Type 1 diabetes during a period of high incidence of the disease (Firman et al., 1985). In another study, approximately 15% of patients with newly diagnosed Type 1 diabetes had evidence of persistent cytomegalovirus infection (Pak, McArthur, Eun, & Yoon, 1988).

It is most likely that a virus that occurs just prior to the onset of symptoms precipitates clinical diabetes rather that the actual autoimmune response, for two reasons: First, various viruses have been shown to be causative agents of diabetes in animal models, isolation of a virus from the pancreas of a child with diabetes has been limited to few case reports of children with coxsackie (Yoon, Austin, Onodera, & Notkins, 1979). Even though mice inoculated with coxsackie from that child developed diabetes, it has now become evident that extensive beta cell damage preceded the onset of the infection (Eisenbarth, 1986).

Second, proponents of the theory that a virus causes Type 1 diabetes point to the temporal relationship of the viral infection and the onset of diabetes. In view of the long prodromal period of Type 1 diabetes, a virus occurring just prior to the onset could not be an initiating factor. The stress of the illness, however, may cause glucose intolerance in a person in whom autoimmune destruction has already started. Therefore, a virus may initiate the autoimmune response, and/or may precipitate the onset of clinical diabetes.

EPIDEMIOLOGY

Age

The incidence of Type 1 diabetes shows a peak onset between 10–14 years of age, approximately 3 times higher than the age group of 0–4 years (Karvonen et al., 2000). There is also a peak presentation occurring at age 5–7 years, coincident with the beginning of school (Karvonen, Tuomilehto, Libmen, & LaPorte, 1993). The difference in age distribution indicates that certain risk factors are more prevalent during certain ages and virtually disappear after age 15. The low incidence of Type 1 diabetes during infancy suggests that there may be protective factors operating in early life (Bennett, 1985).

Gender

In the United States, the incidence of Type 1 diabetes is similar in males and females (Karvonen et al., 2000). This is unlike all other autoimmune diseases that show a large female predominance.

Race

The annual incidence of Type 1 diabetes in white children in the United States is 15 per 100,000/year (Karvonen et al., 1993). Studies of black populations have shown an incidence of Type 1 diabetes ranging from 3.3 in Alabama to 14.3 in Philadelphia (Lipman et al., 2001; Wagenknecht, Roseman, & Alexander, 1989). Data from Hispanic populations of Mexican ancestry have shown a low incidence of Type 1 diabetes (Gay et al., 1989), although Hispanics of Puerto Rican origin have the highest incidence of any racial group in the United States (Lipman, 1993; Lipman et al., 2001).

The most striking difference between whites and blacks in the incidence of Type 1 diabetes is by age group. The risk of developing diabetes in children < 5 years of age is 1.7–2.8 times > in whites than blacks (Lipman, 1993; Lipman et al., 2001; Rewers et al., 1989). In children 10–14 years old, however, some populations of black children develop diabetes 2.5 times more frequently than white children. Various risk factors must be explored to explain the racial differences according to age group.

Place

It has been found that diabetes varies widely between regions, countries, and populations. Incidence rates of Type 1 diabetes have shown that children in China are almost 20 times less likely to develop Type 1 diabetes than children in the United States, and there is a greater than 300-fold difference among countries in the risk of developing Type 1 diabetes. The highest incidence of diabetes occurs in Finland and Sardinia and the lowest is in Venezuela (Karvonen et al., 2000). The variations seem to follow racial and ethnic distribution.

One important design in investigating differences in disease occurrence among populations employs a migration model. Investigation of the descriptive epidemiology of Type 1 diabetes in populations of a common ancestry will greatly contribute to the understanding of the etiology of Type 1 diabetes (Dorman & LaPorte, 1990). European Jews who have migrated to Israel show a low incidence of Type 1 diabetes similar to native Israelis (Laron et al., 1985). The risks of developing Type 1 diabetes among French Canadian and Jewish children were about double and triple those reported from France and Israel respectively (Siemiatycki et al., 1988).

Seasonal Variation

The first data on the seasonality of onset of Type 1 diabetes were presented in 1926 (Adams, 1926) and have attracted much attention. The incidence of

Type 1 diabetes in the United States varies from month to month; it reaches a peak in midwinter, declines sharply during summer, and then rises in the autumn (Drash, 1987). For those who propose that viruses are a risk factor for the development of Type 1 diabetes, it is of interest to note that the pattern of seasonality is reminiscent of those seen in infectious disease. In addition, the rise of incidence in autumn coincides with children's return to school and increased exposure to infection.

DIABETES MANAGEMENT

Changes in diabetes management have resulted from the findings of the Diabetes Control and Complications Trial (DCCT). The DCCT was a 9-year multicenter prospective study of 1500 patients with diabetes who were 13–39 years old at the start of the study. The patients were randomized into an intensive treatment group and a conventional therapy group. Intensive therapy was defined as a minimum of 3 insulin injections per day or the use of an insulin infusion pump. The researchers found that intensive therapy delayed the onset of retinopathy by 62%. Clinically significant neuropathy was reduced by 60% and the development of clinical grade albuminuria was reduced by 56% (Diabetes Control and Complications Trial Research Group, 1993). Because of the results of this study, tighter control is now a goal of diabetes management. However, it is crucial to note that the patients in the intensive therapy group were continuously involved in ongoing education and support in all aspects of diabetes management. That support may have had a significant effect on the diabetes control. In addition, tight control is not recommended for young children because of the serious danger of hypoglycemia (Drash, 1993).

Insulin Therapy

Intensive therapy involves 3 or more injections a day of insulin or insulin delivered by continuous subcutaneous insulin infusion (CSII). Insulin pumps are most often used by school-aged and adolescent children, but have also been used successfully with toddlers (Kaufman, Halvorson, Fisher, & Pitukcheewanont, 1999). When using subcutaneous injections of insulin, a relatively new, quick-acting insulin is often prescribed. Lispro insulin has a peak action of one hr and a duration of 2 hrs. Lispro is proposed for use immediately prior to meals to reduce postprandial hyperglycemia (Anderson et al., 1997). The rapid action also allows for postprandial use in young children with unpredictable carbohydrate or total calorie intake. The dose of Lispro is calculated based on the grams of carbohydrate consumed. Aspart and Novolog are two other rapid-acting insulin products now available.

To optimize diabetes control with subcutaneous injections, it is recommended that children be treated with 3 or more injections of insulin per day. This regimen consists of a mixture of rapid and intermediate-acting insulin (usually NPH) given before breakfast and before dinner. To improve nocturnal glucose control, intermediate-acting insulin is given before bed. The newest insulin developed is glargine, a biosynthetic insulin analog with a prolonged duration of action. Glargine insulin is peakless and has a 24–28 hr duration (Lepore et al., 2000). It is recommended that patients be treated with one injection of glargine at bedtime and premeal injections of rapid-acting insulin. Treatment with glargine has demonstrated less nocturnal hypoglycemia than treatment with NPH and has been approved for children ≥ age 6 (Yki-Jarvinen et al., 2000).

The usual total daily dose averages one unit of insulin per kilogram of body weight. The dose should be adjusted based on previous blood glucose levels. Diluted insulin (e.g., U50 1:1 dilution) may be prescribed for the very young child. This allows for smaller changes in the daily dose and greater ease in drawing up the dose.

Insulin may be injected into the anterior tissue of the upper arm, the anterior and lateral aspects of the thigh, the buttocks, and the abdomen. The site of insulin injections should be varied to prevent atrophy or hypertrophy. Because absorption varies among sites, it is recommended to rotate within one site for 1 week. The abdomen has the fastest rate of absorption, followed by the arms, thighs, and buttocks. Exercise increases the rate of absorption from all injection sites (ADA, 2000).

It is generally suggested that children 9 years of age and older be taught to self-administer insulin. It is crucial that all insulin injections given by school-age and early adolescent children be supervised by an adult. Premature assignment of sole responsibility to the young patient is increasingly recognized as a potential source of poor diabetes control (Follansbee, 1989).

Monitoring Metabolic Control

Blood Testing

The goal of diabetes management for children is maintaining the blood glucose level 80–150 mg/dl 75% of the time, which requires consistent monitoring. Self-monitored blood glucose (SMBG) can be performed by the patient or a family member at home or away from home. The supplies are easily transportable. Hypoglycemia and hyperglycemia are accurately confirmed and the results are immediate and specific. The obvious disadvantage of capillary blood glucose monitoring is the invasive nature of the procedure. Many testing devices have been developed, including some that allow for testing of the forearm, a less sensitive site than the fingertip (McGarraugh, Schwartz, & Weinstein, 2001).

The test strips are analyzed with the use of a glucose meter. The accuracy of the reading depends on the proper use of the test strips and the meter. Testing should be performed at least 4 times each day and in the event of symptoms of hypoglycemia. Encouraging the child to self-test can be a challenge and the nurse will help the parents with different motivating strategies. Test results should be documented and utilized in regulating the insulin dose. Records should be brought to the diabetes appointment to be reviewed by the diabetes team.

Monitors using noninvasive, near-infrared spectroscopy to measure blood glucose across the dermal barrier of the fingertip have been under development for sometime (Robinson et al., 1992). A noninvasive blood glucose device would be a tremendous boon to diabetes management (Mastrototaro, 1998).

Urine Testing

Testing the urine for glucose and ketones is an easy and noninvasive monitoring method. Glucose is not found in the urine until the renal threshold is exceeded—approximately 180 mg/dl, and is, therefore, not a useful tool for maintaining euglycemia. Monitoring for urine ketones is an important component of diabetes management. Urine ketones indicate fatty acid breakdown, which may be present in the event of an illness, a deficiency of insulin, a decreased food intake secondary to starvation, or when a severe hypoglycemic reaction occurs and the body metabolizes fat for energy. A child should test the urine for ketones whenever the blood glucose is 240 mg/dl or higher, or in the event of an illness. Urine ketones in the morning may indicate hypoglycemia during the night, which is followed by a rebound effect called the *Somogyi phenomenon*. Urine ketones in association with vomiting may indicate ketoacidosis and should be handled as an emergency. If ketones do not resolve with treatment with additional insulin at home, the diabetes team should be notified and the child may require an evaluation in the emergency room (Lipman, DiFazio, & Tiffany-Amaro, 1998).

Glycosylated Hemoglobin

Long-term metabolic control should be evaluated by the diabetes team by measuring the child's glycosylated hemoglobin or hemoglobin HbA_{1C}. Glycosylation is the process in which glucose attaches to hemoglobin nonenzymatically, by a slow, mostly irreversible process (Gray, St. Dennis-Feezle, Clark, & Parker, 1993). The life span of the red blood cell molecule is 90–120 days. Increased levels of blood glucose will increase the percentage of hemoglobin that is glycosylated and will reflect the average glucose concentration for the preceding 2–3 months. It is expressed as a percentage of glycosylated hemoglobin. This is an objective manner to assess long-term diabetes control and to assess whether records of blood glucose levels obtained at home are factual.

Nutrition

The goals of nutritional therapy are addressed in the American Diabetes Association's recommendations and principles for people with diabetes mellitus. The goals include: maintaining near normal blood glucose by balancing food intake with insulin and physical activity; achieving optimal serum lipid levels; providing appropriate calories for normal growth and development in children and adolescents; preventing and treating acute complications of Type 1 diabetes and long-term complications; and improving the overall health of the person with Type 1 diabetes through optimal nutrition (ADA, 2001).

Carbohydrate counting is the most commonly used diet of children with diabetes. Grams of carbohydrates are recommended based on age and weight of the child. When consumed with a mixed meal, the type of carbohydrate does not differentially affect the glycemic excursion (Hollenbeck, Coulston, & Reaven, 1998). Because children with diabetes are at risk for cardiovascular disease, as are adults, less than 10% of their daily calories should be from saturated fats (ADA, 2000).

Meal plans are based on individual preferences, culture, and ethnicity. The child's age and developmental level are considered when planning the diet. Because toddlers often have finicky eating habits, their parents become frustrated with the erratic eating patterns because of their fear of hypoglycemia. Lipman, DiFazio, Meers, and Thompson (1989a) recommend that parents offer small frequent meals, rather than large quantities of food at each mealtime. They state that unrealistic expectations can make the dinner table a battleground and that the child may become very manipulative concerning mealtimes and foods. The use of Lispro insulin has greatly decreased the anxiety of mealtime, as insulin may be given postprandially based upon the child's intake.

Preschool and school-age children also have issues related to food and nutrition. At this age, holiday parties, birthday parties, and excursions with peers are common. Lipman and colleagues (1989a) recommend giving the child small gifts instead of candy at Halloween and other holidays. Trading candy for money or other small presents can also be done at holiday times. Sugar-free drinks can be sent with the child to parties or the party food and drinks can be calculated into the child's daily carbohydrate count.

The adolescent may have the most difficulty with the diabetes diet. Peer pressure and the love of junk food can cause great conflict between the adolescent and the parent. To help improve nutrition, a detailed diet history is obtained and the adolescent helps plan the diet. It is important to incorporate as many of the usual adolescent practices as possible, while at the same time maintaining a sound diabetes diet (Lipman, DiFazio, & Tiffany-Amaro, 1998).

Exercise

Exercise is a vital component in the management of the child with diabetes, and offers many benefits. It assists in the utilization of dietary intake and may decrease the amount of insulin that a child requires. Exercise has been shown to decrease lipid levels in persons with diabetes (Durant et al., 1993). The child is instructed to eat a snack prior to exercising. Exercise lasting < 1 hr usually requires a small snack consisting of carbohydrate, whereas more intense exercise or exercise lasting > 1 hr may require more frequent snacks throughout the activity. An insulin adjustment may also be needed if hypoglycemia occurs frequently as a result of the activity (ADA, 2001).

Hypoglycemia can occur during or immediately following a strenuous activity, but it may also occur several hrs after the activity when the child is resting quietly. The family is instructed to check the child's blood sugar after the activity, before bedtime, and sometimes at 2:00 a.m., to prevent hypoglycemia occurring in the middle of the night.

Hypoglycemia

Low blood sugar is a common complication for the child treated with insulin. Hypoglycemia in a child with diabetes is defined as a blood glucose level < 80 mg/dl. Hypoglycemia often occurs if a meal is missed or late, if the insulin dose is too high, or if strenuous physical activity is undertaken without an added snack. Alcohol ingestion, gastroenteritis, and administering excessive insulin can also precipitate hypoglycemia. Alcohol intensifies insulin action and may inhibit gluconeogenesis (Freinkel et al., 1965).

Sympathetic nervous system stimulation and central nervous system depression account for the signs and symptoms of hypoglycemia. The adrenergic signs of hypoglycemia include: diaphoresis, tremulousness, tachycardia, hunger, weakness, pallor, and dizziness. Central nervous symptoms consist of headache, irritability, poor coordination, combativeness, double vision, and confusion. Signs of severe central nervous system depression from hypoglycemia include unconsciousness or convulsions. Since infants are not able to describe their symptoms of hypoglycemia and they usually do not demonstrate the adrenergic symptoms, parents are taught to rely on blood-glucose monitoring and to administer glucose in the form of juice or tubes of decorative cake icing squirted inside the cheek pouch.

Treatment of hypoglycemia is based on the severity of the symptoms. In the case of mild to moderate hypoglycemia, simple carbohydrates are the treatment of choice. Fifteen grams of carbohydrate is the usual treatment. Four ounces of juice or regular soda, glucose tablets, glucose gel, or a small tube of commercially available decorative cake icing can be used. Hypoglycemia resulting in loss of consciousness or a convulsion requires treatment with the administration of glucagon, 0.5–1 mg. Glucagon is a counter-regulatory hormone that stimulates gluconeogenesis, which will increase the blood-glucose level by about 80 mg/dl (ADA, 2001). The child should respond within 10–15 min after the injection has been given. Parents are taught to obtain a blood-glucose level prior to giving the glucagon or immediately after the injection has been given to document true hypoglycemia. Children who do not respond within 15 min should receive emergency medical treatment.

Parents and children are taught the causes, symptoms, and treatment of hypoglycemia. The child is advised to wear an identification tag, especially when away from home. Anyone caring for a child with diabetes must know the signs symptoms and treatment of hypoglycemia. Hypoglycemia is a danger for adolescents who use mood altering drugs that could affect the daily routine of food, insulin, and activity (Lipman et al., 1989b). Alcohol decreases the ability to release glucose into the blood and is likely to cause hypoglycemia (Freinkel et al., 1965).

Diabetes Prevention Trial

A goal of diabetes research is to prevent diabetes in individuals who are at risk. Because of the long prodromal period of diabetes, there is a recently completed study to identify those in whom autoimmune destruction has begun, and an intervention to prevent the development of diabetes. The Diabetes Prevention Trial (DPT) screened consenting first-degree relatives of individuals with Type 1 diabetes. For relatives shown to be at risk through evidence of immune markers and decreased insulin production, there was a randomized clinical trial to determine whether low doses of insulin could prevent diabetes by putting the beta cells at rest. Results of this study showed that low dose insulin did not prevent diabetes (Skyler, 2001).

EPIDEMIC OF TYPE 2 DIABETES

Type 2 diabetes is a disease of hyperglycemia caused by insulin resistance. Within the last 10 years there has been an emerging epidemic of Type 2 diabetes in children. The epidemic is most common in black, Hispanic, and Native American children (Rosenbloom, Joe, & Young, 1999). Risk factors for the development of Type 2 diabetes in youth are similar to the risk factors in adults. The risk factors include obesity and family history of Type 2 diabetes. The epidemic of obesity in youth may be a strong causal factor for Type 2 diabetes. Most children with Type 2 diabetes have a BMI higher than the ninetieth percentile (Neufeld, Raffel, et al., 1998).

Early diagnosis of Type 2 diabetes is crucial. *Acanthosis nigricans* is a sign of insulin resistance and is present in 70–90% of children with Type 2 diabetes (Stuart et al., 1998). It is recognized as velvety, hyperpigmented, leathery patches on the skin, most commonly on the neck, axillae, and groin. A glycosylated hemoglobin should be measured on any child having evidence of acanthosis nigricans.

The major treatment of Type 2 diabetes in children is lifestyle changes consisting of weight loss and exercise. These changes are often difficult in the sociocultural context of the family and must be approached from the family's perspective. Currently, insulin and metformin are the only drugs approved by the Food and Drug Administration for the treatment of Type 2 diabetes in children. Metformin enhances insulin sensitivity. Other oral medications should not be used in children until safety information becomes available (ADA, 2000).

Type 2 diabetes in youth is a major public health problem. Primary prevention includes counseling all children and families about the dangers of obesity and the importance of a healthy diet and exercise program. Interventions and research should focus on the prevention of Type 2 diabetes in youth.

Multidisciplinary Approach to Management

Diabetes is a complex disorder requiring education, support, and collaboration from all members of the diabetes team. Diabetes is unique in that the majority of management tasks and decisions occur in the home. Therefore, it is essential that the child and family be the center of the diabetes team. Self-care and a perception of family control over the disorder are hallmarks of successful diabetes management. Scheduling meal plans and interventions should be based on the activities, priorities, and culture of the family. The individualized approach is crucial.

Members of the diabetes team should include a diabetes nurse educator, a pediatric endocrinologist, dietician, social worker, psychologist, pediatrician, school nurse, and teacher. Frequent communication and periodic team meetings facilitate the sharing of information and the development of flexible management plans. The team must always be mindful that the family and the child are the experts in determining the child's short-term and long-term goals, and the purpose of the other members of the diabetes team is to facilitate and support the actualization of the child's and family's goals.

SUMMARY AND CONCLUSIONS

Insulin-dependent diabetes mellitus is one of the most common chronic illnesses in childhood. It is an autoimmune disorder that occurs in genetically susceptible individuals exposed to still unidentified environmental risk factors. The epidemiology of Type 1 diabetes demonstrates that the incidence of this disorder varies greatly among races, ages, and country of origin. Current research is aimed at preventing Type 1 diabetes in at risk individuals in whom there is evidence of beginning autoimmune distraction.

Type 1 diabetes is a complex disorder. The individual with diabetes attempts to normalize blood glucose levels by regulating insulin dose, diet, and exercise. Because the disorder is so complex, a multidisciplinary team is needed for support, education, and collaboration. Most important, children with diabetes and their families should set goals and diabetes management should be structured so that the children may continue their usual activities.

REFERENCES

Adams, S. F. (1926). The seasonal variation of the onset of acute diabetes. *Archives of Internal Medicine, 37*, 861–864.

American Diabetes Association. (2000). Consensus statement: Type 2 diabetes in children and adolescents. *Diabetes Care, 23*, 381–389.

American Diabetes Association. (2001). American diabetes association clinical practice recommendations 2001. *Diabetes Care, 24*(Suppl. 1), S1–33.

Anderson, J. H., Brunelle, R. L., Koivisto, V. A., Pfutzner, A., Trautmann, M. E., Vignati, L., & Dimarchi, R. (1997). Reduction of postprandial hyperglycemia and frequency of hypoglycemia in IDDM patients on insulin-analog treatment. Multicenter Insulin Lispro Study Group. *Diabetes, 46*, 265–270.

Atkinson, M. A., Maclaren, M. K., Riley, W. J., Winter, W. E., Fisk, D. D., & Spillar, R. P. (1986). Are insulin autoantibodies markers for insulin-dependent diabetes mellitus? *Diabetes, 35*, 894–898.

Bao, M. Z., Wang, J. X., Dorman, J. S., & Trucco, M. (1989). HLA-DQB Non-Asp-57 allele and incidence of diabetes in China and the USA (letter). *Lancet, ii*, 497–498.

Bennett, P. H. (1985). Changing concepts of the epidemiology of insulin-dependent diabetes. *Diabetes Care, 8*(Suppl. 1), 29–33.

Bingley, P. J., Bonfacio, E., & Gale, E. A. M. (1993). Can we really predict IDDM? *Diabetes, 42*, 213–220.

Borch-Johnson, K., Mandrup-Poulsen, T., Zachau-Christiansen, B., Joner, G., Christy, M., Kastrup, K., & Nerup, J. (1984). Relation between breast-feeding and incidence rates of insulin-dependent diabetes mellitus. *Lancet, 2*, 1083–1086.

Bougneres, P. F., Carel, J. C., Castano, L., Boitard, C., Paillard, M., Chaussain, J. L., & Bach, J. F. (1988). Factors associated with early remission of type 1 diabetes in children treated with cyclosporine. *New England Journal of Medicine, 318*, 633–370.

Craighead, J. E. (1978). Current views on the etiology of insulin-dependent diabetes mellitus. *New England Journal of Medicine, 299*, 1439–1445.

Diabetes Control and Complications Trial Research Group. (1993). The effect of intensive treatment of diabetes on the development and progression of long-term complications in insulin-dependent diabetes mellitus. *The New England Journal of Medicine, 329*, 977–986.

Diabetes Epidemiology Research International Mortality Study Group. (1991). International evaluation of cause specific mortality and type 1 diabetes. *Diabetes Care, 14*, 55–60.

Dorman, J. S., & LaPorte, R. E. (1990). Type 1 diabetes epidemiology: Next generation of research. *Diabetes Care, 13*, 184–185.

Drash, A. L. (1987). The epidemiology of insulin-dependent diabetes mellitus. *Clinical and Investigative Medicine, 10*, 432–436.

Drash, A. L. (1993). The child, the adolescent, and the Diabetes Control and Complications Trial (editorial). *Diabetes Care, 16*, 1515–1516.

Durant, R. H., Baranowski, T., Rhodes, T., Gutin, B., Thompson, W. O., Carroll, R., Puhl, J., & Greaves, K. A. (1993). Association among serum lipid and lipoprotein concentrations and physical activity, physical fitness, and body composition in young children. *Journal of Pediatrics, 123*, 185–192.

Eisenbarth, G. S. (1986). Type 1 diabetes mellitus. A chronic autoimmune disease. *New England Journal of Medicine, 314*, 1360–1368.

Faas, S., & Trucco, M. (1994a). The genes influencing the susceptibility to type 1 diabetes in humans. *Journal of Endocrinological Investigation, 17*, 477–495.

Fass, S., & Trucco, M. (1994b). The genes influencing the susceptibility to IDDM in humans. *Journal of Endocrinological Investigation, 17*, 477–495.

Firman, G., Fohlman, J., Frisk, G., Diderholm, H., Ewald, U., Kobbah, M., & Tuvemo, T. (1985). An incidence peak of juvenile diabetes. Relation to Coxsackie B immune response. *Acta Paediatrica Scandinavia, 320*, 14–19.

Fohlman, J., & Friman, G. (1993). Is juvenile diabetes a viral disease? *Annals of Medicine, 25*, 569–574.

Follansbee, D. S. (1989). Assuming responsibility for diabetes management: What age? What price? *Diabetes Educator, 15*, 347–353.

Fox, S. I. (1980). *Human physiology* (2nd ed.). Dubuque, IA: Brown.

Freinkel, N., Arky, R. A., Singer, D. L., Cohen, A. K., Bleicher, S. J., Anderson, J. B., Silbert, C. K., & Foster, A. E. (1965). Alcohol hypoglycemia IV. Current concepts of its pathogenesis. *Diabetes, 14*, 350–361.

Gay, E. C., Hamman, R. F., Carosone-Link, P. J., Lezote, D. C., Cook, M., Stroheker, R., Klingensmith, G., & Chase, H. P. (1989). Colorado type 1 diabetes registry: Lower incidence of type 1 diabetes in Hispanics. *Diabetes Care, 12*, 701–708.

Gepts, W. (1965). Pathologic anatomy of the pancreas in juvenile diabetes mellitus. *Diabetes, 14*, 619–633.

Gerstein, H. C. (1994). Does cow's milk cause type 1 diabetes mellitus? A critical review of the clinical literature. *Diabetes Care, 17*, 13–19.

Gray, D., St. Dennis-Feezle, L., Clark, K., & Parker, S. (1993). Nursing planning, intervention and evaluation for altered endocrine function. In D. Broadwell-Jackson & R. Saunders (Eds.), *Child health nursing: A comprehensive approach to the care of children and their families* (pp. 1459–1535). Philadelphia: J. B. Lippincott Co.

Gundersen, E. (1927). Is diabetes of infectious origin? *Journal of Infectious Disease, 13*, 499–506.

Helgason, T., & Jonasson, M. R. (1981). Evidence for a food additive as a cause of ketosis prone diabetes. *Lancet, 2*, 716–720.

Helgason, T., Ewen, S. W., Ross, I. S., & Stowers, J. M. (1982). Diabetes produced in mice by smoked/cured mutton. *Lancet, 2*, 1017–1022.

Hollenbeck, C. B., Coulston, A. M., & Reaven, G. M. (1998). Comparison of glucose and insulin responses to mixed meals of high-, intermediate-, and low-glycemic potential. *Diabetes Care, 11*, 323–329.

Hyoty, H., Hiltunen, M., Reunanen, A., Leinikki, P., Vesikari, T., Lounamaa, R., Tuomilehto, J., & Akerblom, H. K. (1993). Decline of mumps antibodies in type q (insulin-dependent) diabetic children and a plateau in the rising incidence of type 1 diabetes after introduction of the measles-mumps-rubella vaccine in Finland. Childhood Diabetes in Finland Study Group. *Diabetologia, 36*, 1303–1308.

Karjalainen, J. K. (1990). Islet-cell antibodies as predictive markers for type 1 diabetes in children with high background incidence of disease. *Diabetes, 39*, 1144–1150.

Karjalainen, J. K., Martin, J. M., Knip, M., Ilonen, J., Robinson, B. H., Savilahti, E., Akerblom, H. K., & Dosch, H. M. (1992). A bovine albumin peptide as a possible trigger of insulin-dependent diabetes mellitus. *New England Journal of Medicine, 327,* 302–307.

Karvonen, M., Tuomilehto, J., Libman, I., & LaPorte, R. E. (1993). A review of the recent epidemiological data on the worldwide incidence of type 1 (insulin-dependent) diabetes mellitus. World Health Organization DIAMOND Project Group. *Diabetologia, 36,* 883–892.

Karvonen, M., Viik-Kajander, M., Moltchanova, E., Libman, I., LaPorte, R., & Tuomilehto, J. (2000). Incidence of childhood type 1 diabetes worldwide. *Diabetes Care, 23,* 1516–1526.

Kaufman, D. L., Erlander, M. G., Clare-Salzer, M., Atkinson, M. A., Maclaren, N. K., & Tobin, A. J. (1992). Autoimmunity to two forms of glutamate decarboxylase in insulin-dependent diabetes mellitus. *Journal of Clinical Investigation, 89,* 283–292.

Kaufman, F. R., Halvorson, M., Fisher, L., & Pitukcheewanont, P. (1999). Insulin pump therapy in type 1 pediatric patients. *Journal of Pediatric Endocrinology & Metabolism, 12*(Suppl. 3), 759–764, UI: 20091712.

LaPorte, R. E., Matsushima, M., & Chang, Y. F. (1995). Prevalence and incidence of insulin-dependent diabetes. In *Diabetes in America* (2nd ed., pp. 37–47). Bethesda, MD: National Institutes of Health, No. 95-1468.

Laron, A., Karp, M., & Modan, M. (1985). The incidence of insulin-dependent diabetes mellitus in Israeli children and adolescents 0–20 years of age: A retrospective study, 1975–1980. *Diabetes Care, 9*(Suppl. 1), 24–28.

Lendrum, R., Walker, G., & Gamble, D. R. (1975). Islet-cell antibodies in juvenile diabetes mellitus of recent onset. *Lancet, 1,* 880–882.

Lipman, T. H. (1993). The epidemiology of type 1 diabetes in children 0–14 years of age in Philadelphia. *Diabetes Care, 16,* 922–925.

Lipman, T. H., DiFazio, D. A., Meers, R. A., & Thompson, R. L. (1989a). A developmental approach to diabetes in children: Birth through preschool. *American Journal of Maternal Child Nursing, 14,* 225–229.

Lipman, T. H., DiFazio, D. A., Meers, R. A., & Thompson, R. L. (1989b). A developmental approach to diabetes in children: Schoolage through adolescence. *American Journal of Maternal Child Nursing, 14,* 330–332.

Lipman, T. H., DiFazio, D. A., & Tiffany-Amaro, J. (1998). Health challenge: Alterations in endocrine status. In V. Bowden, S. Dickey, & S. Greenberg (Eds.), *Children and their families: A continuum of care* (pp. 1803–1860). Philadelphia: Saunders.

Lipman, T. H., Jawad, A. F., Murphy, K., Katz, L. L., Fuchs-Simon, J., Tuttle, A., & Thompson, R. (2001). Incidence of type 1 diabetes in Philadelphia is higher in black than white children from 1995–2000: Epidemic a misclassification? *Diabetes, 30*(Suppl. 2), A39.

Mastrototaro, J. (1998). Clinical results from a continuous glucose sensor multi-center study. *Diabetes, 47,* A61.

McGarraugh, G., Schwartz, S., & Weinstein, R. (2001). Glucose measurements using blood extracted from the forearm and the finger. *TheraSense, Inc.,* 1–7.

Neufeld, N. D., Raffel, L. J., Landon, C., Chen, Y. D., & Vadheim, C. M. (1998). Early presentation of type 2 diabetes in Mexican-American youth. *Diabetes Care, 21,* 80–86.

Norris, J. M., Dorman, J. S., Rewers, M., & LaPorte, R. E. (1987). The epidemiology and genetics of insulin-dependent diabetes mellitus. *Archives of Pathology and Laboratory Medicine, iii,* 905–909.

Olmos, P., A'Hern, R., Heaton, D. A., Millward, B. A., Risley, D., Pyke, D. A., & Leslie, R. D. (1988). The significance of the concordance rate for type 1 (insulin-dependent) diabetes in identical twins. *Diabetologia, 31,* 747–750.

Pak, C. Y., McArthur, R. G., Eun, H. M., & Yoon, J. W. (1988). Association of cytomegalovirus infection with autoimmune type 1 diabetes. *Lancet, ii,* 14.

Raffel, L. J., & Rotter, J. H. (1985). The genetics of diabetes. *Clinical Diabetes, 3,* 490–54.

Rewers, M., Stone, R. A., LaPorte, R. E., Drash, A. L., Becker, D. J., Walczak, M., & Kuller, L. H. (1989). Poisson regression modeling of temporal variation in incidence of childhood insulin-dependent diabetes mellitus in Allegheny County, Pennsylvania and Wielkopolska, Poland, 1970–1985. *American Journal of Epidemiology, 129,* 569–581.

Robinson, M. R., Eaton, R. P., Haaland, D. M., Koepp, G. W., Thomas, E. V., Stallard, B. R., & Robinson, P. L. (1992). Noninvasive glucose monitoring in diabetic patients: A preliminary evaluation. *Clinical Chemistry, 38,* 1618–1622.

Rose, N. R., & Mackay, I. R. (Eds.). (1985). *The autoimmune diseases.* Orlando: Academic Press.

Rosenbloom, A. L., Joe, J. R., Young, R. S., & Winter, W. E. (1999). Emerging epidemic of type 2 diabetes in youth. *Diabetes Care, 22,* 345–354.

Scheuner, M. T., Raffel, L. J., & Rotter, J. I. (1997). Genetics of diabetes. In K. G. M. M. Alberti, P. Zimmet, & R. A. Defronzo (Eds.), *International textbook of diabetes mellitus* (2nd ed., pp. 37–55). New York: Wiley.

Siemiatycki, J., Colle, E., Campbell, S., Dewar, R. A., Aubert, P., & Belmonte, M. M. (1988). Incidence of diabetes in Montreal by ethnic group and by social class and comparisons with ethnic groups living elsewhere. *Diabetes, 37,* 1096–1102.

Skyler, J. (2001). Results of the DPT-1. [Presented at the 61st Annual Meeting of the American Diabetes Association, June 24, 2001.]

Spencer, K. M., Tarn, A., Dean, B. M., Lister, J., & Bottazzo, G. F. (1984). Fluctuating islet-cell autoimmunity in unaffected relatives of patients with insulin-dependent diabetes. *Lancet, 1,* 764–766.

Stuart, C. A., Gilkison, C. R., Smith, M. M., Bosma, A. M., Keenan, B. S., & Nagamani, M. (1998). Acanthosis nigricans as a risk factor for non-insulin dependent diabetes mellitus. *Clinical Pediatrics, 37,* 73–79.

Sultz, H. A., Hart, B. A., & Zielezny, M. (1975). Is mumps virus an etiologic factor in juvenile diabetes mellitus? *Journal of Pediatrics, 86,* 654–656.

Tarn, A. C., Thomas, J. M., Dean, B. M., Ingram, D., Schwarz, G., Botazzo, G. G., & Gale, E. A. (1988). Predicting insulin-dependent diabetes. *Lancet, I,* 868–878.

Thorsby, E., & Ronningen, K. S. (1993). Particular HLA-DQ molecules play a dominant role in determining susceptibility or resistance to type 1 (insulin-dependent) diabetes mellitus. *Diabetologia, 36,* 371–377.

Volpe, R. (Ed.). (1985). *Autoimmunity and endocrine disease.* New York: Dekker.

Wagener, D. K., Kuller, L. H., & Orchard, T. J. (1982). Pittsburgh Diabetes Mellitus Study: Secondary attack rate in families with insulin-dependent diabetes mellitus. *American Journal of Epidemiology, 115,* 868–878.

Wagenknecht, L. E., Roseman, J. M., & Alexander, W. J. (1989). Epidemiology of type 1 diabetes in black and white children in Jefferson County, Alabama, 1979–1985. *Diabetes, 38,* 629–633.

Waife, S. D. (Ed.). (1980). *Diabetes mellitus* (9th ed.). Indianapolis: Lilly Research Laboratories.

Yki-Jarvinen, H., Dressler, A., & Ziemen, M. (2000). Less nocturnal hypoglycemia and better post-dinner glucose control with bedtime insulin glargine compared with bedtime NPH insulin during insulin combination therapy in type 2 diabetes. *Diabetes Care, 23,* 1130–1136.

Yoon, J., Austin, M., Onodera, T., & Notkins, A. L. (1979). Virus-induced diabetes mellitus: Isolation of a virus from the pancreas of a child with diabetic ketoacidosis. *New England Journal of Medicine, 300,* 1173–1179.

CHAPTER 3

Juvenile Idiopathic Arthritis

Diane Carol Hudson-Barr and Sally A. Lambert

C hildhood arthritis was first described by George Frederic Still in 1896 as a systemic disease presenting with fever, arthritis, splenomegaly, and enlarged lymph nodes (Davidson, 2000). Since that time, much disagreement existed over the classification and terminology of chronic arthritis in childhood. The lack of a universally accepted classification system led to the formation of an international task force that proposed (1995) and revised (1997) a new classification of the childhood arthritis disorders (Davidson, 2000). The terms *juvenile rheumatoid arthritis* (JRA, North America) and *juvenile chronic arthritis* (JCA, Europe) have been replaced with the internationally accepted *juvenile idiopathic arthritis* (JIA).

Juvenile idiopathic arthritis is the most frequently occurring major connective tissue disease in children and is a major cause both of functional disability and eye disease leading to blindness in children (Cassidy & Petty, 1995). JIA is currently defined as (1) continuously active arthritis (2) involving one or more joints (3) for a minimum of 6 weeks (4) in a child who is younger than 16 years of age, and (5) who has no other demonstrable disease. In addition, at least two of the following conditions are present: swelling, pain, or limited joint motion. Other names for JIA include juvenile arthritis and, when the onset is marked by a systemic illness, Still's disease.

INCIDENCE

The incidence rate of JIA is approximately 10/100,000 (Davidson, 2000; Cassidy & Petty, 1995). This is similar to those for juvenile diabetes mellitus and all forms of childhood cancer. Estimates suggest 250,000 American children have been diagnosed with JIA (Schaller, 1997). The peak incidence is from infancy to 3 years of age, and from 7–11 years of age (Cassidy & Petty, 1995). Females are affected twice as often as males.

ETIOLOGY

Generally considered to be autoimmune in origin, the etiology of JIA is not known (Murray, Thompson, & Glass, 1997). It has been suggested that JIA is a syndrome of diverse etiologies instead of one single disease (Cassidy & Petty, 1995). Four etiologies have been suggested: (1) immunogenetic predisposition or immunologic deficiency, (2) latent viral infection, (3) trauma, and, (4) stress. It is rare for more than one family member to have JIA, yet an increased incidence of polyarthritis in other family members has been documented. In addition, certain human leukocyte antigen (HLA) subtypes have been associated with specific characteristics of JIA, and other subtypes have been hypothesized to protect against the development of JIA. Chronic arthritis occurs frequently in children with immunologic deficiencies like immunoglobulin and complement component deficiencies (Petty, Cassidy, & Tubergen, 1977). Many viral diseases, like rubella, parvovirus, mycobacteria, and Epstein-Barr virus, have joint inflammation associated with the course of the virus and have been suggested as potential triggers of JIA (Petty, 1997). Yet, the causal relationship between these infections and the development of JIA has not been proven (Petty, 1997). The onset of JIA has followed physical trauma to an extremity, although it is unclear whether the trauma calls attention to an already involved joint or precipitates the disease (Cassidy & Petty, 1995). Psychological stress is well documented as a common occurrence in families of children with JIA, but it is not clear whether the stress precedes or results from the diagnosis of JIA (Cassidy & Petty, 1995). Researchers continue to explore the association between the immune system, infection, trauma, stress, and JIA.

DIAGNOSING JIA

The diagnosis of JIA is challenging; the presence of juvenile arthritis can also be associated with other rheumatic and connective tissue diseases (Cassidy & Petty, 1995; Schaller, 1997). Differential diagnoses include: systemic

lupus erythematosus (SLE), scleroderma, spondyloarthropathies, inflammatory bowel disease, and rheumatic fever. Seven types of onset have typically
been used for classification: (1) systemic, (2) oligoarthritis, (3) polyarthritis
with negative rheumatoid factor, (4) polyarthritis with positive rheumatoid
factor, (5) psoriatic, (6) ethesitis related arthritis, and (7) other (not meeting
criteria for 1–6) (Davidson, 2000).

A typical presentation of the child with JIA might include increased
irritability, joint-guarding posture, refusal to crawl or walk, low grade fever,
and fatigue. Many children also exhibit anorexia, weight loss, and failure to
grow (Cassidy & Petty, 1995). General symptoms of JIA include morning
stiffness and night pain. Children may not be able to specify any more than
"it hurts." Careful questioning of the caregiver and careful observation of
the child are essential to detect the signs of JIA.

Systemic Arthritis

Systemic onset of JIA occurs in about 10% of children with the disease.
Classic symptoms include high spiking fevers associated with a 2–5 mm
erythematous macular migratory rash most commonly located on the trunk,
proximal extremities, or over pressure areas (Cassidy & Petty, 1995). Systemic
JIA most often occurs in children younger than 5 years of age, with an
equal incidence between the genders. Extraarticular manifestations occur in
approximately 20% of the cases, including hepatosplenomegaly, enlarged
lymph nodes, and pericarditis. Systemic involvement may precede overt
development of arthritis by weeks or months (Cassidy & Petty, 1995). Approximately half those diagnosed with systemic arthritis have a chronic and
destructive arthritis course.

Oligoarthritis (Pauciarticular) Arthritis

Children diagnosed with oligoarthritis JIA have arthritis in four or fewer
joints. This is the mildest form of JIA and accounts for approximately 50%
of those diagnosed. The knees and ankles are commonly affected. Hips are
usually spared. Involvement may be asymmetrical. Eighty percent of the
cases are females diagnosed between 1–3 years of age. Children with oligoarthritis JIA have less significant joint disease. Children in this subgroup
are at risk of developing chronic uveitis that can lead to blindness (Tibbitts,
1994). More recent data suggest that the prevalence of uveitis has decreased
to about 20% of those affected with oligoarthritis (Davidson, 2000).

Polyarthritis Arthritis (Rheumatoid Positive and Negative)

Within 6 months of the onset of symptoms, five or more joints are involved. Initially, however, fewer joints may have been involved. Approximately 40% of children diagnosed with JIA have polyarthritis onset. Approximately 10% of those with polyarthritis onset test positive for rheumatoid factor (Davidson, 2000). Large and small joints are involved; commonly knees, wrists, elbows, and ankles. A symmetrical pattern is often seen. Soft tissue swelling, osteoporosis, and articular changes occur in 90% of those having the polyarthritis JIA for at least 10 years. Radial deviation of fingers, loss of motion in the cervical spine in as many as 60% of those diagnosed, and as high as a 30-fold increase in the incidence of lower spine scoliosis has been reported (Cassidy & Petty, 1995). In addition, temporomandibular joint (TMJ) involvement leading to loss of normal bite or micrognathia have been reported in as many as 50% diagnosed with JIA (Ronchezel et al., 1995). Chronic uveitis occurs in < 5% of the children with polyarthritis involvement. Systemic signs, including low-grade fever, slight to moderate hepatosplenomegaly, and lymphadenopathy may occur, but are not as acute or as persistent as those affected by the systemic form. Onset is either before age 2, or during the teenage years. Joint destruction and growth disturbances may occur.

Psoriatic Arthritis

Arthritis and psoriasis and at least two of the following characterize the child with psoriatic arthritis: (1) nail pitting or onycholysis, (2) family history of psoriasis in a first degree relative, or dactylitis (Davidson, 2000). Psoriatic arthritis was rarely categorized before the 1997 international classification was accepted; therefore the incidence data is unavailable. Children with psoriatic arthritis may have polyarticular or oligoarthritic disease.

Enthesitis Related Arthritis

A new diagnostic category for children having both arthritis and enthesitis (inflammation at the insertion of tendons into bones) and at least two of the following: (1) presence of HLAB27, (2) family history of HLAB27 disease, (3) sacroiliac joint tenderness and/or inflammatory spinal pain, (4) onset of arthritis in a boy over 8 years of age, or (5) acute anterior uveitis (Davidson, 2000). This categorization recognizes that those children with HLAB27 positive disease behave differently than those who are not positive. The majority of this group is older boys presenting with asymmetrical large joint arthritis in the lower limbs.

Other Arthritis

The final category includes children who do not fit easily into the first six categories. Experts expect that as the understanding of JIA increases, new diagnostic categories will be developed, and fewer children would be categorized here (Davidson, 2000).

DISEASE COURSE IN JIA

Joint inflammation results in hypertrophy of the synovium and hyperplasia of the synovial lining layer (Cassidy & Petty, 1995). Synovial tissues are edematous and hyperemic, often accompanied by hyperplasia of the vascular endothelium, and infiltration of plasma cells and lymphocytes. Articular cartilage, and later contiguous bone, become progressively eroded and destroyed (Hamalainen, 1994). These tissue changes result in joint contracture, joint damage, and altered growth (American Juvenile Arthritis Organization [AJAO], 1996). Fibrous ankylosis (abnormal immobilization/fixation of the joint) is fairly common in the hips and knees (Tibbitts, 1994). The rate of joint destruction for all types is slower in children with JIA than adults having rheumatoid arthritis. The period of time that damage is reversible is also prolonged with JIA. (See Cassidy & Petty [1995] for a more detailed physiological description.)

ECONOMIC IMPACT

Allaire, De Nardo, Szer, Meenan, and Schaller (1992) attempted to quantify the economic impact of JIA for 70 families receiving care in the Boston area. The cost of the disease was explored from three perspectives: (1) the direct cost for health care (inpatient/outpatient medical care and JIA illness-related nonmedical expenses), (2) family expenses meeting the special health care needs of children with JIA (out of pocket expenses not paid/reimbursed by insurance, nonmedical expenses, and loss of salary related to helping the child obtain necessary health care), and (3) special school service costs. Direct costs to the family averaged $7905 annually: $1717/child for inpatient care, $5700/child for outpatient care, and $488/child for nonmedical care. Although 96% of the families had private insurance, additional costs paid by family that were not reimbursed included $1524/year (or 19% of the direct costs). Five percent of the family income was spent on the management of their child's JIA. In addition, 20% of the children (14/69) required special school services costing, on the average, $7135/year. The out-of-pocket expenses incurred by the families in this study were comparable to those experienced by families in the eastern Pennsylvania (McCormick, Stemmler, & Athreya, 1986) and southern Ohio areas (Plummer, Rennebohm, & Koebel, 1990). The national direct cost of JIA in the United States in 1989, calculated from an incidence of 36,000 cases (0.5 cases/1000), was estimated to be $285 million (Allaire et al., 1992). The cost of special education requirements to the community was estimated to be an additional $52 million. Outpatient medical care for JIA was more expensive per family than that for cystic fibrosis ($5700/year versus $3170/year). Professional service costs for JIA were only a little less than those for childhood cancer ($5231/year versus $3956/year) (Allaire et al., 1992). Thus, from the data, it is clear that the economic impact of JIA on the family, community, and national economy is substantial.

CLINICAL EVALUATION AND TREATMENT

The goal of comprehensive treatment of the child diagnosed with JIA is to assess adequately his or her physical, mental, and social state, and, to develop a plan of care with the child and family that ensures as normal as possible mental, physical, and social growth (Hamalainen, 1994).

Diagnostic Tests

Joint counts are completed to identify the number and location of the affected joints. Laboratory assays include serum, urine, and synovial fluid tests (see Table 3.1 for specific tests and results).

Radiological examination evaluates soft tissue swelling, atrophy, loss of bone density, periosteal new bone formation, and bone fractures resulting from generalized osteoporosis (Cassidy & Petty, 1995; Tibbitts, 1994). The cervical spine also is evaluated for changes including fusion of upper apophyseal joints (Cassidy & Petty, 1995). The extent of soft tissue or bone involvement can be identified using radionucleid scanning, thermography,

TABLE 3.1 Laboratory Tests

Laboratory test	Results with JIA	Special considerations
Hemoglobin (HgB)	Mild to severe anemia: 7–10 g/dL (usually normal in children with pauciarticular JIA)	
White blood cells (WBC)	15,000–25,000/mm^3 with polyarticular 30,000–50,000/mm^3 with systemic JIA (usually normal in children with pauciarticular JIA)	
Erythrocyte sedimentation rate (ESR)	Pauciarticular JIA: 20–60 mm/hr Polyarticular JIA: 20–60 mm/hr Systemic JIA: 100 mm/hr or greater	Useful in acute phase of diagnosis; occasionally helpful monitoring medication regime; may be elevated for months or years.
C-reactive protein (CRP)	Seropositive	Detected before elevated ESR. Disappears with inflammation suppressed by steroids/salicylates.
Rheumatoid factor (RF)	Seropositive (about 4% positive at onset; only 10–20% of patients diagnosed with JIA are positive)	Less common in children diagnosed with JIA than adults diagnosed with rheumatoid arthritis.
Antinuclear antibody (ANA)	Seropositive (about 40% will be seropositive; 65–85% of those with pauciarticular onset and uveitis are seropositive.)	Critical in initial diagnostic workup as indicator of those to watch closely for developing uveitis.
Associated human leukocyte antigens (HLA)	Pauciarticular JIA: DR5, DR8 Polyarticular JIA: DR4, DR8, Dqw4, DR5, DR6, DR1 Systemic JIA: DR4, DR8, DR5	
Synovial fluid analysis	Increased WBC count; low complement activity; usually RF positive	Elevated WBC not always correlated with degree of clinical activity; complement levels not uniformly depressed in all children diagnosed with JIA
Urinalysis	Usually normal	Proteinuria may be associated with a fever; intermittent hematuria suggestive of mild glomerulitis, drug toxicity, or the development of other diseases, like SLE.

(Tibbitts, 1994; Wallach, 1983)

ultrasonography, computed tomography (CT), and magnetic resonance imaging (MRI).

Management

Several challenges affect the process and content of developing a plan of care. These factors have to do with the disease/condition itself, as well as with its treatment, including: (1) current antiinflammatory and immune therapies are imprecise in children (Shaller, 1997); (2) the prognosis is unpredictable, therefore, it is difficult to identify children most in need of early, aggressive therapy (Tibbitts, 1994); (3) the chronic inflammatory course of the disease necessitates treatment plans that last for years that must be acceptable to the child, family, and health care team; and, (4) the recognition by the child and family that total elimination of the signs and symptoms of JIA may not be possible (Cassidy & Petty, 1995). Critical members of the treatment team include: the child, the parents, the pediatric rheumatologist, nurses, physical and occupational therapists, social workers, and orthopedic surgeons. Consultation also may be required from psychologists, nutritionists, and school teachers.

Pharmacologic Management

Drug therapy is the cornerstone of the medical management of the child diagnosed with JIA. The goals of pharmacologic therapy are to provide analgesia/relief of pain, to suppress inflammation, control synovitis until spontaneous remission occurs, diminish cartilage destruction, and prevent deformities (Davidson, 2000; Rose & Doughty, 1992). The specifics of drug therapy are reviewed in Table 3.2.

Nonsteroidal Antiinflammatory Drugs

Nonsteroidal antiinflammatory drugs (NSAIDs) are used for their antiinflammatory, antipyretic, and analgesic actions. Therapy is started with aspirin. Research conducted by the Paediatric Rheumatology Collaborative Study Group suggest 65% of children who are going to respond to NSAID therapy do so within 4 weeks of beginning therapy (Cassidy, 1999). Late responders may take up to 12 weeks to respond; therefore a 3-month trial is recommended before switching to tolmetin, naproxen, or ibuprofen (Cassidy, 1999; Cas-

TABLE 3.2 Pharmacologic Agents Used in the Management of JIA

Generic/proprietary name Dosage/route/frequency	Side effects/contraindications/indications to stop therapy	Laboratory tests to monitor
NSAIDs		
Acetylsalicylic acid (aspirin, bufferin, ascriptin) 75–100 mg/kg/day divided QID PO	Chewing aspirin associated with gingival inflammation & erosion of biting surfaces of teeth (child must swallow; use liquid form or have dentist coat teeth)	Desirable serum level of salicylate is 15–30 mg/dL (2 hours after morning dose)
Give with meals or with milk to decrease gastric irritation	Complaints of stomach pain may indicate gastric injury (buffered/enteric coated may be preferred; or magnesium choline salts of salicylate can be useful)	Baseline tests include CBC, AST, ALT, BUN and creatinine, then every 3–4 months
> 100 mg/kg/day usually results in toxicity	Anorexia	AST, ALT, transaminase enzymes may be intermittently elevated in as many as 50%
Fever usually responds within 1 to 4 weeks of beginning therapy; antiarthritic action generally achieved in 2–4 weeks	Increased shin bruising, epistaxis	of those on therapeutic levels (do not discontinue aspirin with transient increases)
	Can develop hepatitis, most frequently with toxic serum levels	
	Due to potential association between salicylates and Reye's syndrome, NSAIDs should be stopped in any vomiting sick child who may have varicella/influenza	
	Contraindicated in children with glucose-6-diphosphate deficiency, pyruvate kinase deficiency, hemophilia, von Willebrand's disease, and those on anticoagulant therapy	
Naproxyn (Aleve, anaprox, naprosyn) 10–20 mg/kg/day given BID/TID; maximum dose is 1250 mg); PO Suspension form available	See aspirin Dermal toxicity (pseudoporphria) more common in fair-skinned children and with sun exposure	See aspirin

(continued)

55

TABLE 3.2 *(continued)*

Generic/proprietary name Dosage/route/frequency	Side effects/contraindications/indications to stop therapy	Laboratory tests to monitor
Ibuprofen (Advil, motrin, nuprin) 30–50 mg/kg/day given TID/QID (maximum dose is 3200 mg); PO Suspension form available	See aspirin Liquid dose should be 45 mg/kg/day because of differential absorption of the 2 drug enantiomers (mirror image components of the medication)	See aspirin
Indomethicin (indocin) 1–4 mg/kg/day given TID/QID (maximum dose is 200 mg); PO	Nausea, dyspepsia, headache, and dizziness Also, see aspirin	See aspirin
Tolmetin sodium (tolectin) 15–30 mg/kg/day given QID (maximum dose is 1800 mg); PO	See aspirin	See aspirin
Immunosuppressives		
Methotrexate (Rheumatrex) PO dosing of 5–10 mg/m²/wk; Give on empty stomach with clear liquids, 1 hr before breakfast May use liquid injectable orally	(see below)	

TABLE 3.2 *(continued)*

Generic/proprietary name Dosage/route/frequency	Side effects/contraindications/indications to stop therapy	Laboratory tests to monitor
Immunosuppressives (continued) NSAIDs may interfere with protein binding/excretion of this drug; keep dosage constant during therapy	Less toxic than with adults: gastric ulceration, headache, diarrhea, interstitial pneumonitis, alopecia, dermatitis, cirrhosis (rare) Leukopenia, bone marrow suppression Malignancy mutagenic effects Sterility, amenorrhea Folic acid (1 mg/day) usually administered along with MTX If used in combination with NSAIDs, keep NSAID dose constant due to potential drug interactions with albumin-binding	Dosage adjusted based on 1 & 24 hr blood levels obtained after 1 month of therapy Baseline CBC with differential, albumin, BUN, hepatitis screen, U/A, renal/liver pulmonary function, eye exam, & chest X-ray CBC, LFTs and U/A every 4 weeks initially, then every 8 weeks
SAARDS Antimalarial: hydroxychloroquine sulfate (Plaquenil) 5–7 mg/kg/day (maximum 600 mg) Onset of action takes several months Take with food	Bone marrow suppression, dermatitis, gastrointestinal irritation If corneal deposition observed, decrease dosage Discontinue with any signs of retinopathy (effects are cumulative) If no observable response in 6 months, may change to another SAARD	Baseline ophthalmologic examination; follow-up every 4 months (children 4–7 years are difficult to test for color vision—not use with this age group)
Gold salts: auranofin (Ridaura) Initial test dose of 5 mg IM 0.75–1.0 mg/kg/week Maximum dosage 50 mg	Microscopic hematuria; dermatitis; loose stools in 10% of children Absolute contraindications with severe leukopenia, neutropenia, proteinuria, exfoliative dermatitis Typically on maintenance at least 6 months Relapse may be delayed up to 3 months after stopping therapy Wean dose slowly after documented articular improvement	Baseline CBC, WBC with differential, U/A, liver and renal function studies CBC and U/A every 2 weeks Biochemistry every 6 weeks

(continued)

TABLE 3.2 *(continued)*

Generic/proprietary name Dosage/route/frequency	Side effects/contraindications/indications to stop therapy	Laboratory tests to monitor
Gold salts: gold sodium Thiomalate (Myochrysine) Initial test dose of 5 mg Weekly injection gradually increased to 0.75–1 mg/kg/week (maximum dosage 50 mg) Usually 20 weeks of therapy; after satisfactory improvement/remission, administer every 2 weeks for 3 months; then every 3 weeks for 3 months; then every 4 weeks	Signs of toxicity: stomatitis, dermatitis; bone marrow suppression, hematuria, proteinuria Those with systemic onset JIA may have greater risks of reactions (neutropenia, DIC) Discontinue temporarily with decreased WBC < 4500/mm^3 or ANC decreased by 50%; eosinophilia; proteinuria; clinical signs of toxicity	Baseline CBC, WBC with differential, U/A, liver and renal function studies Liver and renal function labs every 6 weeks CBC and U/A before each administration
Antimalarial: sulfasalazine (Azulfidine) Begin with 10 mg/kg/day, once a day; gradually increase frequency over 4–6 weeks for total of 30–60 mg/kg/day given TID/QID; PO Maximum dosage: 2000 mg/day Take with food/milk	Gastric irritation, diarrhea Oral ulcerations Dermatitis (including Steven-Johnson Syndrome); hypersensitivity reactions Mood changes Bone marrow suppression Male infertility Contraindicated in children with porphyria, glucose-6-phosphate dehydrogenase; not indicated in children with a known sensitivity to sulfa/salicylates or with impaired hepatic/renal function	Baseline laboratory tests include hepatic function Follow CBC, U/A, biochemistry once a month

TABLE 3.2 *(continued)*

Generic/proprietary name Dosage/route/frequency	Side effects/contraindications/indications to stop therapy	Laboratory tests to monitor
After initial treatment period, decrease maintenance dose to 25 mg/kg/day		
Use suspension with younger child; enteric-coated with older children		
Clinical response seen within 6–8 weeks, but a minimum trial of 3 months is recommended		
D-pencillamine (Cuprimine, Depen)	Drug-induced lupus	Baseline CBC, U/A, biochemistry
Same indications as gold salts; do not use while administering gold	Dermatitis, rash, pruritis	CBC, U/A weekly
Begin at 3 mg/kg/day; increase in two increments over 8–12 weeks time to 10 mg/kg/day (< 750 mg/day maximum dose)	Nausea, vomiting, loss of taste Thrombocytopenia Proteinuria Bone marrow suppression Nephrotoxicity	Biochemistry every 6 weeks
Administer early in the morning on an empty stomach	Signs of toxicity are not necessarily dose-related It may take 9 months–3 years for maximum effectiveness to be achieved	

TABLE 3.2 *(continued)*

Generic/proprietary name Dosage/route/frequency	Side effects/contraindications/indications to stop therapy	Laboratory tests to monitor
Glucocorticosteriods		
0.1–1 mg/kg/day (dosage may be as high as 2 mg/kg/day given TID;maximum dose 40 mg); PO	Cushing's syndrome, growth suppression, osteopenia, fractures, increased susceptibility to infection; watch for signs of hypokalemia & hyperglycemia; decrease caloric intake; may restrict sodium; may administer antacids to combat dyspepsia	
Given as single, morning dose (divided with more severe disease)	Do not administer live virus immunizations (OPV, MMR); recommend varicella zoster immune globulin within 48 hrs of exposure in any nonimmune child on steroid therapy	
Increase dosage with stress, serious infection, traumatic injury; taper dose when discontinuing		
Triancinolone hexacetonide 5–40 mg intraarticular in one of a few inflamed joints	Do not give more than three times in a single joint during a three month period	
Effect may last weeks/months	Recurrent injections can lead to infection, crystal-induced synovitis, calcification, and osteoporosis	
Methylprednisolone 10–30 mg/kg/pulse; i.v.	Electrolyte and fluid imbalance	Continuous cardiorespiratory monitoring during pulse therapy and several hours afterwards
Single dose or three pulses administered on alternate days Effects last 3–6 weeks	Cardiac arrhythmias	
Steroid eye drops In combination with mydriatic drug	May result in Cushing's syndrome	Supervised by experienced opthalmologist

(Cassidy, 1999; Cassidy, 1993; Giannini & Cawkwell, 1995; Rose & Doughty, 1992; Tibbitts, 1994) sidy & Petty, 1995). Schaller (1997) recommended a separate clinical trial of at least two NSAIDs to determine whether or not optimal clinical response has been achieved. Optimal clinical response is demonstrated by the best balance between preventing exacerbation of symptoms, tolerating the amount of pain experienced, and the ability to complete activities of daily living with limited assistance with the lowest dose of medication and minimization of side effects. Fifty to 70% of those diagnosed with JIA respond to treatment with NSAIDs alone (Cassidy & Petty, 1995; Tibbitts, 1994). Therapy is continued for 2 years after symptoms have disappeared.

Immunosuppressive Agents

Once a week, low dose methotrexate (MTX) has been demonstrated to be the next most effective drug when the child does not respond to NSAIDs (Cassidy, 1999). Methotrexate (MTX) is the only agent used with children with JIA that has rarely demonstrated oncogenicity (one case of Hodgkins disease reported in 1998) (Onel, 2000) and has not found to be a cause of sterility. MTX is believed to create anti-inflammatory action by affecting T and B lymphocytes, and by suppressing the rheumatoid factor (Rose & Doughty, 1992). It also may inhibit the action of interleuken-1. Effectiveness is usually noted after 2–3 months of treatment. Relapse has been noted as late as 36 months after cessation of MTX, leading Cassidy (1999) to suggest that treatment should continue as long as 1–2 years after remission has been achieved.

Slow Acting Antirheumatic Drugs

The slow acting antirheumatic drugs (SAARDs) include antimalarial drugs, gold salts, d-penicillamine, and sulfasalazine (Cassidy & Petty, 1995). Once the second-line therapy after NSAIDS, the SAARDs are currently added to therapy when the use of NSAIDs and MTX are not enough (Cassidy, 1999). Hydroxychloroquine, an antimalarial drug, has been a useful adjunct in the treatment of the child aged 8 years or older with JIA. Hydroxychloroquine is believed to inhibit DNA/RNA synthesis, stabilize lysosomes, and to interfere with prostaglandin synthesis (Rose & Doughty, 1992). The mechanism of action of gold salts is unknown, but is thought to inhibit macrophage differentiation, and to decrease human leukocyte antigen (HLA) expression (Rose & Doughty, 1992). It takes several months for observable clinical change. Gold salts may hold hope for the actual improvement of the course of the disease (Tibbitts, 1994). Gold salts are indicated for the child with polyarthritis onset who has been unresponsive to the more conservative medication regime. Indications for the use of d-penicillamine are the same as those for gold. The two drugs should not be administered together as part of the medication regime. In a review of 18 studies using sulfasalazine (SSZ) with JIA, Brooks (2001) found SSZ demonstrated drug-associated benefit in all subtypes of JIA. It has been found to be relatively safe and demonstrates a clinical response within 6–8 weeks (Cassidy & Petty, 1995).

Glucocorticosteroids

Steroids have been used to provide a therapeutic bridge, covering for the latency of action of other medications used in the treatment of JIA (Rose & Doughty, 1992). The challenge in using steroids is to balance the goal of management of persistent inflammation that restricts normal motion and activity, with the risks of toxicity. Small doses of oral steroids have been found to improve morning stiffness when treatment with NSAIDs is inadequate. Intravenous steroid pulse therapy may be used to treat more severe manifestations of JIA. Opthalmic steroids may be used in treatment of uveitis. Local treatment of acutely inflamed joints may be accomplished by the use of intraarticular steroids.

Additional Second-Line Medications

A variety of other pharmacologic interventions have been reported. Limited success has been achieved using cyclosporine to block the production of interleukin-2 (cytokine). Monthly administrations of intravenous human immune globulin (IVIG) have been effective at improving systemic symptoms of JIA, but not as effective in controlling arthritis lasting longer than one year (Roifman, 1995).

EXPERIMENTAL TREATMENTS. Few of the approaches studied with adults diagnosed with arthritis have been explored in children diagnosed with JIA. Newly developed drugs, like cyclooxygenase-2 inhibitors (COX-2 inhibitors), and novel therapies like stem cell transplantation may offer hope for those children (Onel, 2000). Etanercept, which is believed to bind with tumor necrosing factor and therefore protects the synovia and joints from being destroyed, has been trialed in the management of JIA with moderate success (Onel, 2000). Because etanercept has been associated with increases in severe infections, cautious use of this agent is recommended until more is known about its effects.

Surgical Intervention

Surgery is the treatment of last resort in JIA (Tibbitts, 1994). The goals of surgery include: (1) delay/prevention of joint destruction and closure of the epiphysis, (2) prevention or correction of deformities, (3) decrease pain, and, (4) maintain joint growth and motion. Prophylactic surgical treatments include soft tissue releases, joint synovectomies, and tenosynovectomies. As the child enters adolescence and young adulthood, the importance of a well thought out plan for reconstructive surgery may be critical to promoting optimal functional status. Procedures include closure of the growth plate, joint resections, and surgical reformation of joints after growth has been completed (Hamalainen, 1994; Tibbitts, 1994).

Nonpharmacologic Treatments

Along with the pharmacologic management of the child diagnosed with JIA, the following interventions are critical to providing a treatment plan that addresses physical, emotional, and social issues for the child and family.

Exercise and Rehabilitation

A reduction in aerobic activity and decreased physical activity may occur due to stiffness, pain, and chronic fatigue. Making exercise a part of the routine is therefore important for the child diagnosed with JIA. A balanced plan of local and generalized rest of the affected joints is beneficial to many children. A convenient time to provide increased rest is either at night or shortly after school. Children are adept at determining their own level of activity and should be encouraged to take an active role in regulating their involvement. Encouraging normal play and involvement in exercise programs the child finds enjoyable is also important. Help the family identify activities that are practical, inexpensive, oriented to the child, and foster the child's independence (Singsen, 1995). Tricycle/bike riding, low impact dance, and swimming are most often helpful and avoid putting weight on involved joints (Singsen, 1995). Basketball and some forms of gymnastics put increased levels of stress on inflamed weight-bearing joints and are less desirable (Cassidy & Petty, 1995).

Physical and Occupational Therapy

The goal of physical and occupational therapy interventions is to maintain overall function and to prevent deformities. Children tend to immobilize joints in flexion position to reduce tension on the joint and decrease joint pain. This classic posture is often referred to as *guarding*. Physical and occupational therapies focus on maintaining and restoring functional range of motion in each joint, strengthening muscles around joints, and allowing joints to remain in positions of function. Exercising the affected joint(s) and splinting are the mainstay of these therapies. Preventing malpositioning or aiding in long-term correction of joint deformity can be accomplished through the use of splints. Maintaining reduction of contractures can be promoted with gentle stretching and the use of resting splints. Physical and occupational therapy both promote optimal functioning in the child diagnosed with JIA.

Clinical assessment tools have been developed to assess functional status and identify what physical activities the child can perform. The Juvenile Arthritis Functional Assessment Scale (JAFAR) (Lovell et al., 1989), the Juvenile Arthritis Functional Assessment Report for Children and Parents questionnaires (JAFAR-C, JAFAR-P) (Howe et al., 1991), and the Juvenile Arthritis Functional Status Index (JASI) (Wright et al., 1996) demonstrated significant correlations with rheumatology measures like joint count, grip strength, pain scores, and adult functional status measures. These four tools show great promise for evaluating the functional status of the child with JIA. In addition, The Juvenile Arthritis Quality of Life Questionnaire (JAQQ) has been developed to assess physical and psychosocial function and a variety of physical symptoms in children diagnosed with JIA and juvenile spondyloarthritides (Duffy, Arsenault, Paquin, & Strawczynski, 1997).

Education and Adjustment of the Child and Family

Education is a central component of the management of JIA. A consistent education program that stresses explaining the nature of JIA, identifying reasonable expectations during the initial therapy, and the course of disease must be initiated early in the management plan. *Understanding Juvenile Rheumatoid Arthritis: A Health Professional's Guide to Teaching Children and Parents* is an excellent resource, produced by the Arthritis Foundation (1987). Encouraging the family members to write down questions they might have and providing opportunities for telephone contact are beneficial. A list of community resources available for the family is reviewed in Table 3.3. Preliminary work on the development of a questionnaire to assess perceived

TABLE 3.3 Family Resource List

Organization	Purpose	Address	Telephone
American Juvenile Arthritis Organization	Arthritis Foundation council dedicated to serving special needs of children, teens, and young adults with childhood rheumatic disease & their families	Internet: http://www.arthritis.org/events/ajao_programs_services.asp Email: ajao@arthritis.org	(800)-283-7800 (404)-965-7514
National Center for Youth with Disabilities	Chronic illnesses, disabilities and transition to adult life	NCND, University of Minnesota, Box 721, 420 Delaware Street SW, Minneapolis, MN 55455 Internet: www.peds.edu/centers/ihd/ncyd.html	
National Parent Network on Disabilities	National presence/voice for parents of children, youths, and adults with disabilities	1130 17th Street, NW, Suite 400, Washington, DC 20036 Internet: www.npnd.org/ Email: npnd@mindspring.com	(202) 463-2299
National Information Center for Children and Youth with Disabilities	Links people with common concerns for children and youth with disabilities	Box 1492 Washington, DC 20013-1492 Internet: www.nichcy.org	(800) 695-0285 (answered live 9:30a–6:30p EST)
Parent to Parent Programs	Parent group located in most states to support parents of a child with special needs	The Beach Center, University of Kansas, 3136 Haworth Hall, Lawrence KS 66045 Internet: www.beachcenter.org/ (choose Families) Email: beach@dole.lsi.ukans.edu	The Beach Center of Families and Disability at (785) 864-7600

TABLE 3.3 (continued)

Written resource	Address	Telephone
Kids Get Arthritis Too!	Hugh MacMillian Rehabilitation Centre, 350 Rumsey Road, Toronto, ON M4G 1R8	(416) 425-6220 1-800-363-2440 (tollfree in Canada); (416) 425-6591 (fax)
JRA & Me: A Fun Workbook	Rocky Mountain Juvenile Arthritis Center, National Jewish Center for Immunology and Respiratory Medicine, 1400 Jackson Street, Denver, CO 80206	
When Your Student Has Arthritis	Arthritis Foundation, PO Box 19000, Atlanta GA 30326 or The Arthritis Society, 250 Bloor St. E., Suite 901, Toronto, ON M4W 3P2	

Webpage with general rheumatology links on the internet: www/edae.gr/reumatology.html (Note: no 'h' in rheumatology is correct).

ability to manage JIA among adolescents and their parents has been described by Andre, Hedengren, Halgenber, and Stenstrom (1999). The questionnaire enables evaluation of four underlying dimensions: medical issues, exercise, pain, and social support.

Successful management of the child's disease depends in a large part on the parents being able to provide the prescribed care. A qualitative study by Jerrett (1994) explored the changes reported by parents ($N = 19$) as they adjusted to being the parent of a child with JIA. Parents had to make adjustments in their role as they provided care to the child. Additions to the parental role included providing physical therapy, administering medications, ensuring the consistent use of splints, transportation to appointments, and routine visits to the health care providers. Parents reported struggling with causing their children pain during therapy. Learning to control time and becoming more organized were also crucial to successful adaptation to parenting a child diagnosed with JIA.

Parents also reported feeling they needed to take charge and have the final say about their child's plan of care, including having the ability to challenge the medical authorities (Jerrett, 1994). Bartholomew, Koenning, Dahlquist, and Barron (1994) suggest compliance with the medical regimen for children with JIA is challenging due to the complexity, the time-consuming nature, and the intrusiveness in family lifestyle.

Involvement of School Agencies

The physical differences and limitations in activity may make attendance at school difficult and complicated. Regardless, encouraging children to attend school is critical to their social and mental development. Challenges facing the child with arthritis include: difficulty with writing assignments/tests, severe joint stiffness while at school, difficulty in carrying books to/from school (Spencer, Fife, & Rabinovich, 1995), inadequate time to get from one class to another, trouble turning handles/opening locks, inability to participate fully in physical education class, increased absenteeism, poor self-image, and decreased social interaction (Bartholomew et al., 1994). Education' sessions with the child's principal, school nurse, and teacher may facilitate a smoother transition for the child and family.

Public laws 94–142, 99–458, and subsequent amendments established that children with a disabling or chronic illness are entitled to early intervention and the same educational opportunities as other children. These Public laws also establish a mechanism for legal recourse if children are denied these opportunities. Children with JIA are eligible for evaluation of special education services in every state (Spencer et al., 1995). If the child's condition interferes with the ability to function in school, the child is eligible for special services from the particular state department of special education or equivalent (Spencer et al., 1995). The special services are individually determined on a case-by-case basis and are outlined in the Individual Education Plan (IEP) document. The IEP identifies services necessary for the child to improve his/her education experiences.

ADDITIONAL CONCERNS FOR THE CHILD DIAGNOSED WITH JIA

Chronic Uveitis

Chronic uveitis most frequently occurs in young girls with oligoarthritis onset who are ANA seropositive. Chronic uveitis is primarily a chronic inflammation affecting the iris and ciliary body. Onset is usually insidious and asymptomatic—less than 2% report redness, pain, or decreased visual acuity (Cassidy & Petty, 1995). A routine eye exam should be performed at diagnosis and frequently during the early years of JIA. An opthamologist should supervise the treatment of chronic uveitis.

Growth Retardation

Growth retardation is characteristic in children with JIA. Children with long-term JIA rarely achieve full stature. Henderson, Lovell, and Gregg (1992) reported up to one third of those children diagnosed with JIA have heights less than the fifth percentile for age. Growth disturbances may result from the primary disease process, malnutrition, or drug effects (Purdy, Dwyer, Holland, Goldberg, & Dinardo, 1996). The development of secondary sexual characteristics is often delayed. Common areas of growth arrest include the jaw and extremities. Micrognathia may result from failure of normal development in one or both temporomandibular growth centers, or contiguous involvement of the cervical spine. Early in active disease, accelerated development of ossification centers in the knee may result in leg length discrepancies, whereby the involved leg grows longer (Cassidy & Petty, 1995). Later in the course of the disease, premature ossification of the epiphysis can result in short stature and brachydactyly (Cassidy & Petty, 1995).

Malnutrition

Like all children, the child with JIA needs to follow a well-balanced diet that includes a variety of foods. Children with JIA are at risk for developing inadequate protein-calorie and nutrient intake, drug-nutrient interactions, anorexia, obesity, and/or mechanical feeding difficulties (Purdy et al., 1996). Many children with JIA have persistent or intermittent anorexia, and have been found to consume only 50–80% of the recommended daily allowances for their needs as determined by indirect calorimetry (Henderson & Lovell, 1991). Children with poor appetites need to be encouraged to eat higher caloric/nutrient-rich foods like peanut butter sandwiches, cheese and crackers, shakes, and nuts and seeds (Purdy et al., 1996). Evaluation by a dietitian is recommended for all children diagnosed with JIA.

CHRONIC PAIN AND JIA

Pain is a consistent feature in all types of JIA and is a major predictor of physical and psychological outcome (Lovell & Walco, 1989). Recent studies of the pain associated with JIA suggest most children report mild to moderate pain (Shanberg, Lefebvre, Keefe, Kredich, & Gil, 1997). Clinicians involved in the care and treatment of children with JIA have a responsibility to assess and treat the chronic pain associated with this disease.

The pain experienced by children with JIA is most frequently due to the joint inflammation component of the disease process. The degree of pain experienced is dependent on the amount of tissue damage and inflammation. The rich network of nerve fibers and nerve endings in the tissues of the musculoskeletal system are most likely activated by those factors associated with infection: heat, mechanical pressure, and the chemical mediators of infection (Lovell & Walco, 1989). In addition, periarticular soft tissue edema and synovial effusions cause swelling, pain with motion, and tenderness (Cassidy & Petty, 1995). The pain of JIA may be acute, as that occurring at the onset of the disease, and/or chronic, as that which occurs over time with chronic inflammation. The untreated pain of JIA may result in school absences, decreased mobility and activity, and decreased social interaction with family members and others.

The assessment and management of arthritis pain in children is challenging in part because many of the children newly diagnosed with JIA are under 3 years of age (Vandvik & Hoyeraal, 1993). At this stage of development, the child may not have the words or experiences to describe and communicate the pain experience. The inability to describe the pain sensations poses problems in the assessment and treatment of the toddler's pain. Pain at this age may best be evaluated in terms of the child's activity level and ability to participate in developmentally appropriate activities. Numerous studies have demonstrated the validity of parental report of the child's pain (Jaworski, Bradley, Heck, Roca, & Alarcon, 1995; Thompson, Varni, & Hanson, 1987; Walco, Varni, & Ilowite, 1992). The toddler with pain from JIA might decrease activity, favor an affected limb or show other behavioral signs that might indicate their discomfort. Parents are aware of the toddler's activity level and special pain words, such as "ouchy" or "booboo." In fact, many parents notice changes in the child not easily observed by a health professional. Thus, parental evaluation of the child's pain is an integral component of the assessment of the child's pain experience.

Beales and colleagues (1983) attempted to account for the child's developmental level and ability to report pain. They interviewed 39 children with JIA and asked them how their joints felt. Young children (6–11 years) reported their joints had an aching sensation and older children (12–17 years) reported sharp or burning pain. All the children rated the sensations as unpleasant. When given the developmentally appropriate words, children were able to describe their pain. Jaworski and colleagues (1995) developed an observation method for assessing pain in children with JIA. In their sample of children (6–11 years), the pain behaviors most frequently observed included guarding, passive rubbing, rigidity, and simple flexion. The highest pain scores on a visual analogue scale positively correlated with total frequency of observed behaviors ($r = .50$) and disability levels ($r = .64$).

There are several instruments with established reliability and validity that can be used to assess acute pain in children and youth. Chronic pain, including that associated with JIA, has different effects requiring different forms/types of assessment. The development of observational tools to measure the chronic pain of JIA in toddlers must be considered in the future.

Older children and adolescents are able to describe and quantify their pain. Words chosen by school-age children to describe JIA pain include hurting, warm, uncomfortable, and stinging (Abu-Saad & Uiterwijk, 1995). The school-age child has an increased ability to think in abstract terms, has some understanding of cause and effect, and is able to attach meaning to a painful experience. Self-report of the chronic pain experience becomes easier in this age group.

Varni and Thompson developed a Pediatric Pain Questionnaire (PPQ) to measure chronic and recurrent pain in children (Varni, Thompson, & Hanson,

1987; Varni et al., 1996). The PPQ was designed to be sensitive to the cognitive developmental conceptualizations of children. Recognizing the complex nature of pediatric chronic pain, Varni and Thompson proposed a multidimensional assessment of chronic childhood pain. The intensity of the pain is addressed on a visual analog scale and body outline. Sensory, affective, and evaluative qualities of pain are evaluated by asking the child to select terms that best describes their pain. Child, adolescent, and parent forms of the PPQ have been developed and tested. Early studies (Varni et al., 1987; Varni & Walco, 1988) demonstrated positive correlations between children's and parents' (r = .72) and children and physicians' pain assessment (r = .65). Based on Varni's work, Abu-Saad and Uiterwijk (1995) developed the Pediatric Pain Assessment Tool (PPAT) designed to be culturally and developmentally sensitive. They tested this tool on a group of children with JIA in the Netherlands and demonstrated correlations between the child and parent's pain rating (r = .77) and the child and physician's pain ratings (r = .43). The work of Abu-Saad and Uiterwijk confirmed that of Varni and colleagues that children can accurately describe their chronic pain.

The Pain Coping Questionnaire (PCQ) has been developed to measure coping with pain in children and adolescence (Reid, Gilbert, & McGrath, 1998). Eight subscales measure coping strategies previously reported in the literature. These 8 subscales represent 3 scales of coping: approach (directly dealing with the pain), problem-focused (disengaging from the pain), and emotion-focused avoidance (expressing emotions associated with the pain). After being tested on healthy children and adolescents, a sample of children/ adolescents experiencing recurrent pain were studied. Two groups of subjects were included: children and adolescents with arthritis (*n* = 28) or headaches (*n* = 48). Parents of those enrolled also completed the PCQ from their child's perspective. A low correlation between child and parent responses was found; this may be due to the fact that many of the coping strategies are internal ones and not visible to the parent. Therefore, the tool most likely would not be accurate if completed by the parent. Findings in this study were consistent with others that have addressed coping with general stressors and pain in children (Reid et al., 1998). The PCQ can be used with children as young as 8 years of age and takes approximately 15 min to complete. Assessment of children's pain coping strategies can be evaluated using the PCQ.

Psychological variables have a considerable influence on the child's chronic pain. Ross and colleagues (1993) found a significant relationship ($R^2 = 0.43$, p < .001) between family conflict/harmony and maternal distress and the child's pain. Higher self-report of pain for children and adolescents was associated with higher depressive symptoms, higher anxiety, and lower self-esteem (Varni et al., 1996). Because the intensity and duration of pain and disease activity change over time, chronic pain measurement should not be based on a one time self-report (Ross et al., 1993; Thompson et al., 1987; Varni et al., 1987). The assessment should consider the child's pain over time (at least the previous week), and include sensory and affective components. To obtain a true assessment of the child's pain observation, self-report, and assessment of other pertinent factors contributing to the child's overall health status are necessary. Pain is not a unidimensional concept and cannot be treated as such.

There is some evidence that children with chronic pain have lower pain thresholds than healthy children. Walco and colleagues (1990) investigated the relationship between pain threshold levels and chronic pain, and found children with JIA had significantly lower pain thresholds, concluding that recurrent pain may sensitize children. Hogeweg and colleagues (1995) also demonstrated decreased pain thresholds in children with JIA. They surmised that nocioception from inflamed joints in patients with JIA may have established changes in the peripheral and central nociceptive processing system in JIA. The results of these studies suggest it is important to treat the pain associated with JIA with therapeutic interventions, such as relaxation techniques or the use of transcutaneous electrical nerve stimulation (TENS), that reduce the activity of the sympathetic nervous system. Chronic pain may increase the child's sensitivity to other pain experiences so that the treatment of acute pain for these children may need to be increased or modified.

The goal of treatment is to achieve a level pain control that allows the child to function and thus, accomplish necessary developmental tasks. Pharmacological treatment of JIA also contributes to pain management by helping control the swelling and joint inflammation. Children are taught to conserve energy, use their joints wisely to reduce stress, and maintain regular exercise (Kuis, Heijnen, Hogeweg, Sinnema, & Helders, 1997). Proper rest and diet is taught. The use of heat, cold, and massage may also decrease pain and stiffness. Devices such as splints and braces can stabilize joints, provide strength, and reduce pain and inflammation (Arthritis Foundation, 1987).

It is important to foster healthy coping skills for children with chronic pain. Varni and colleagues (1996) described pain coping strategies used by children with JIA to include cognitive self-instruction (tell self to be brave, pretend doesn't hurt so much); problem solving (go to bed, ask for medication, lie down); distraction (watch TV, play a game); and seeking social support (ask for hug, play with friends). They also found that children who used cognitive refocusing experienced lower pain and fewer depressive symptoms, suggesting that active cognitive concentration away from the pain may result in lower perceived pain. Schanberg and colleagues (1997) found teaching coping strategies that increase the child's perception of pain self-efficacy and pain control result in improved quality of life for children diagnosed with JIA.

Teaching children cognitive behavioral strategies to relieve chronic pain also may have some merit. The goal of these strategies is to modify the subjective response to pain. Relaxation, imagery, and self-hypnosis have proven useful in the treatment of children with other painful medical conditions such as cancer, migraines and procedure-related pain (Kuttner, 1989; Olness, MacDonald, & Uden, 1987; Zeltzer & LeBaron, 1982). Children who learn these techniques have the added benefit of mastery and may be able to utilize these strategies in other aspects of their life. One study by Walco and colleagues (1992) demonstrated the successful use of progressive muscle relaxation, guided imagery and meditative breathing to reduce the pain intensity experienced by children with JIA. Teaching children strategies that promote productive coping and mastery may improve long-term adaptation.

Parents have considerable influence on the child's reaction to pain. Kuttner (1996) offers guidance to parents in managing a child with chronic pain at home. Recognizing that the child's pain can lead to frustration, fatigue, and continued readjustment for the child and family, Kuttner suggested that parents establish a management plan that includes a support system, allowing other trusted persons to care for the child, and treating the pain promptly. The child becomes the authority and participates in the treatment plans. Parents are encouraged to seek health care providers that encourage and enhance both parents' and child's coping skills and those who include them as equal partners in the planning the treatment.

OUTCOME FOR THE CHILD DIAGNOSED WITH JIA

There is no uniformly accepted symptom, sign, or supplementary test that predicts which children with JIA will do well or poorly, even within the individual subgroups (Vandvik, Fagertun, & Hoyeraal, 1991). Seventy to ninety percent of children with JIA make a satisfactory recovery without serious disability (Cassidy & Petty, 1995; Tibbitts, 1994). Children with systemic JIA are the most prone to develop life-threatening, even fatal complications. Children with oligoarthritis JIA tend to do best in relation to joint disease but have worse outcomes with regard to uveitis. Cassidy (1993) reported 10% of children with JIA enter adulthood with significant functional disability. Others (Wallace & Levinson, 1991) have suggested the duration of disease is a valid predictor of limitation: 31% diagnosed with JIA for at least 10 years have severe functional limitation whereas 47% having the disease for at least 20 years exhibit severe functional limitation.

Prediction of physical and psychosocial outcomes in JIA was studied in 84 children by Vandvik and colleagues (1991). Biological and psychological factors that predicted the disease course were identified. Maternal distress and the child's behavioral problem score, along with age at onset, months of disease duration, disease severity, presence of rheumatic disease in the family, thrombocytes, and ESR, correctly classified 81% of the patients as improved or unchanged/worse when compared with physician assessment of status. Vandvik and Eckblad (1991) found no relationship between maternal distress, child behavior problems, and chronic family difficulties and the child's severity of illness during the early stages of the disease.

The severity of the child's disease, as rated by the parent and the physician, has been shown to affect the child's psychological adjustment (Daltroy et al., 1992). Teenagers with recent onset disease were found to have poorer social competence scores on the Child Behavior Checklist than population norms. Baildam and colleagues (1995) found increased physical disability was not associated with increased psychological reactions: children 7–16 years of age had a median score on a self-concept scale similar to that of a healthy population. Sixty percent of the subjects who had been diagnosed with JIA for a mean of 20 years were employed, and 38% believed their arthritis had no impact on their ability to form relationships.

CONCLUSIONS

The successful treatment and management of JIA is dependent on a multidisciplinary approach. As a chronic disease, JIA affects the child and family in all areas of their life. The child may have limitation in function that affects activities and thus interferes with the child's life in the areas of social development and school, and the child might suffer from both acute and chronic pain. The family may need to learn many new treatments and may need to restructure their lives and activities to meet the needs of the child. The research on the short- and long-term effects of JIA is minimal and conflicting.

It is clear that both positive and negative outcomes occur. Clinicians caring for these children should be aware of the current treatment strategies, promote a healing atmosphere, and support the child's comfort and the parent's caregiving abilities (Spurrier & White, 1995).

THE FUTURE

Children with JIA will continue to require the input of a variety of disciplines and resources to meet their needs. The importance of designing care models to provide services to these children in a cost-effective manner must take priority. Health care providers must be able to critically evaluate the cost-benefit ratio of resources and outcomes along the continuum of care for children with JIA.

Additional research is needed on children with JIA and their families. Increased rigor is needed in the scientific investigation of treatment and management of JIA. Increasing sample size, multisite studies, and longitudinal samples are some examples of needed methodological improvements. Expanded areas for development include: (1) the impact of disease severity on the child's ability to transition to adulthood, (2) system factors that promote health of the child, (3) research focusing on health outcomes and quality of life in chronic illness, and (4) research on pain measurement and management, with continuing emphasis on exploring the impact of alternative interventions such as relaxation, imagery, and hypnosis on the pain experience of the child with JIA.

REFERENCES

Abu-Saad, H. H., & Uiterwijk, M. (1995). Pain in children with juvenile arthritis: A descriptive study. *Pediatric Research, 38*(2), 194–197.

Allaire, S. H., De Nardo, B. S., Szer, I. S., Meenan, R. F., & Schaller, J. G. (1992). The economic impacts of juvenile arthritis. *Journal of Rheumatology, 19*, 952–955.

American Juvenile Arthritis Organization. (1996). Available on internet: www.arthritis.org/events/ajaoprogramsservices.asp

Andre, M., Hedengren, E., Hagelberg, S., & Stenstrom, C. H. (1999). Perceived ability to manage juvenile chronic arthritis among adolescents and parents: Development of a questionnaire to assess medical issues, exercise, pain, and social support. *Arthritis Care Research, 12*(4), 229–237.

Arthritis Foundation. (1987). *Understanding juvenile rheumatoid arthritis: A health professional's guide to teaching children and parents.*

Baildam, E. M., Holt, P. J. L., Conway, S. C., & Morton, M. J. S. (1995). The association between physical function and psychological problems in children with juvenile chronic arthritis. *British Journal of Rheumatology, 34*(5), 470–477.

Bartholomew, L. K., Koenning, G., Dahlquist, L., & Barron, K. (1994). An educational needs assessment of children with juvenile arthritis. *Arthritis Care and Research, 7*(3), 136–143.

Beales, J. G., Holt, P. J., Keen, J. H., & Mellor, V. P. (1983). The child's perception of the disease and experience of pain in juvenile chronic arthritis. *Journal of Rheumatology, 10*, 61–65.

Brooks, C. D. (2001). Sulfasalazine for the management of juvenile rheumatoid arthritis. *The Journal of Rheumatology, 28*(4), 845–853.

Cassidy, J. T. (1993). What's in a name? Nomenclature of juvenile arthritis. A North American view. *Journal of Rheumatology Supplement*, Oct; *40*, 4–8.

Cassidy, J. T. (1999). Medical management of children with juvenile rheumatoid arthritis. *Drugs, 58*(5), 831–850.

Cassidy, J. T., & Petty, R. E. (1995). *Textbook of pediatric rheumatology* (3rd ed.). Philadelphia: W. B. Saunders.

Davidson, J. (2000). Juvenile idiopathic arthritis: A clinical overview. *European Journal of Radiology, 33*, 128–134.

Daltroy, L. H., Larson, M. G., Eaton, H. M., Partridge, A. J., Pless, L. B., Rogers, M. P., & Liang, M. H. (1992). Psychosocial adjustment in juvenile arthritis. *Journal of Pediatric Psychology, 17*(3), 277–289.

Duffy, C. M., Arsenault, L., Duffy, K. N., Paquin, J. D., & Strawczynski, H. (1997). The Juvenile Arthritis Quality of Life Questionnaire—development of a new responsive index for juvenile rheumatoid arthritis and juvenile spondyloarthritides. *Journal of Rheumatology, 24*(4), 738–746.

Giannini, E. H., & Cawkwell, G. D. (1995). Drug treatment in children with juvenile arthritis: Past, present, and future. *Pediatric Clinics of North America, 42*(5), 1099–1125.

Hamalainen, M. (1994). Surgical treatment of juvenile arthritis. *Clinical and Experimental Rheumatology, 12*(Suppl. 10), 107–112.

Henderson, C. J., & Lovell, D. J. (1991). Nutritional aspects of juvenile arthritis. *Rheumatic Disease Clinics of North America, 17*, 403–413.

Henderson, C. J., Lovell, D. J., & Gregg, D. J. (1992). A nutritional screening test for use in children and adolescents with juvenile arthritis. *The Journal of Rheumatology, 19*, 1276–1281.

Hogeweg, J. A., Kuis, W., Oostendorp, R. A. B., & Helders, P. J. M. (1995). General and segmental reduced pain thresholds in juvenile chronic arthritis. *Pain, 62*, 11–17.

Howe, S., Levinson, J., Shear, E., Hartner, S., McGirr, G., Schulte, M., & Levinson, J. (1991). Development of a disability measurement tool for juvenile arthritis. *Arthritis Rheumatology, 34*, 873–880.

Jaworski, T. M., Bradley, L. A., Heck, L. W., Roca, A., & Alarcon, G. S. (1995). Development of an observation method for assessing pain behaviors in children with juvenile arthritis. *Arthritis & Rheumatism, 38*(8), 1142–1151.

Jerrett, M. D. (1994). Parents' experience of coming to know the care of a chronically ill child. *Journal of Advanced Nursing, 19*(6), 1050–1056.

Kuis, W., Heijnen, C. J., Hogeweg, J. A., Sinnema, G., & Helders, P. J. M. (1997). How painful is juvenile chronic arthritis? *Archives of Disease in Childhood, 77*, 451–453.

Kuttner, L. (1989). Management of young children's acute pain and anxiety during invasive medical procedures. *Pediatrician, 16*, 39–44.

Kuttner, L. (1996). *A child in pain: How to help, what to do.* Washington, DC: Hartley & Marks.

Lovell, D. J., Howe, S., Shear, E., Hartner, S., McGirr, G., Schulte, M., & Levinson, J. (1989). Development of a disability measurement tool for juvenile rheumatoid arthritis: The Juvenile Arthritis Functional Assessment Scale. *Arthritis Rheumatology, 32*, 1390–1395.

Lovell, D. J., & Walco, G. A. (1989). Pain associated with juvenile arthritis. *Pediatric Clinics of North America, 36*, 1015–1027.

McCormick, M. C., Stemmler, M. M., & Athreya, B. H. (1986). The impact of childhood rheumatic diseases on the family. *Arthritis and Rheumatology, 29*, 872–878.

Murray, K., Thompson, S. D., & Glass, D. N. (1997). Pathogenesis of juvenile chronic arthritis: Genetic and environmental factors. *Archives of Disease in Childhood, 77*, 530–534.

Olness, K., MacDonald, J., & Uden, D. (1987). Prospective study comparing propanolol, placebo, and hypnosis in management of juvenile migraine. *Pediatrics, 79*(4), 593–597.

Onel, K. B. (2000). Advances in the medical treatment of juvenile rheumatoid arthritis. *Current Opinion in Pediatrics, 12*, 72–75.

Petty, R. E. (1997). Viruses and childhood arthritis. *Annals of Medicine, 29*, 149–152.

Petty, R. E., Cassidy, J. T., & Tubergen, D. G. (1977). Association of arthritis with hypogammaglobulimenia. *Arthritis Rheumatology, 20*, 441.

Plummer, M. E., Rennebohm, R., & Koebel, S. M. (1990). *The distribution and amount of direct and indirect costs for rheumatic diseases in children attending a multidisciplinary comprehensive clinic.* Available from M. E. Plummer, Arthritis Program, Ohio Department of Health, P. O. Box 118, Columbus, OH, 43266.

Purdy, K. S., Dwyer, J. T., Holland, M., Goldberg, D. L., & Dinardo, J. (1996). You are what you eat: Healthy food choices, nutrition, and the child with juvenile arthritis. *Pediatric Nursing, 22*(5), 391–398.

Reid, G. J., Gilbert, C. A., & McGrath, P. J. (1998). The pain coping questionnaire: Preliminary validation. *Pain, 76*, 83–96.

Roifman, C. M. (1995). Use of intravenous immune globulin in the therapy of children with rheumatological diseases. *Journal of Clinical Immunology, 15*(Suppl 6), 42–51.

Ronchezel, M. V., Hilario, M. O., Goldenberg, J., Lederman, H. M., Faltin, K., de Azevedo, M. F., & Naspitz, C. K. (1995). Temporomandibular joint and mandibular growth alterations in patients with juvenile rheumatoid arthritis. *Journal of Rheumatology, 22*, 1956–1961.

Rose, C. D., & Doughty, R. A. (1992). Pharmacological management of juvenile arthritis. *Drugs, 43*(6), 849–863.

Ross, C. K., Lavigne, J. V., Hayford, J. R., Berry, S. L., Sinacore, J. M., & Pachman, L. M. (1993). Psychological factors affecting reported pain in juvenile arthritis. *Journal of Pediatric Psychology, 18*(5), 561–573.

Schaller, J. G. (1997). Juvenile rheumatoid arthritis. *Pediatrics in Review, 18*(10), 337–349.

Schanberg, L. E., Lefebvre, J. C., Keefe, F. J., Kredich, D. W., & Gil, K. M. (1997). Pain coping and pain experience in children with juvenile chronic arthritis. *Pain, 73*, 181–189.

Singsen, B. H. (1995). Physical fitness in children with juvenile arthritis and other chronic pediatric illnesses. *Pediatric Clinics of North America, 42*(5), 1035–1050.

Spencer, C. H., Fife, R. Z., & Rabinovich, C. E. (1995). The school experience of children with arthritis: Coping in the 1990s and transition into adulthood. *Pediatric Clinics of North America, 42*(5), 1285–1298.

Spurrier, K., & White, P. (1995). You are not alone: Advocacy for children & young adults with rheumatic diseases. *Pediatric Clinics of North America, 42*(5), 1299–1309.

Thompson, K. L., Varni, J. W., & Hanson, V. (1987). Comprehensive assessment of pain in juvenile arthritis: An empirical model. *Journal of Pediatric Psychology, 12*(2), 241–255.

Tibbitts, G. M. (1994). Juvenile arthritis: Old challenges, new insights. *Postgraduate Medicine, 96*(2), 75–87.

Vandvik, I. H., & Eckblad, G. (1991). Mothers of children with recent onset of rheumatic disease: Associations between maternal distress, psychosocial variables, and the disease of the children. *Development and Behavioral Pediatrics, 12*(2), 84–91.

Vandvik, I. H., Fagertun, H., & Hoyeraal, M. (1991). Prediction of short term prognosis by biopsychosocial variables in patients with juvenile rheumatic diseases. *Journal of Rheumatology, 18*, 125–132.

Vandvik, I. H., & Hoyeraal, H. M. (1993). Juvenile chronic arthritis: A biobehavioral disease: Some unsolved questions. *Clinical and Experimental Rheumatology, 11*, 669–680.

Varni, J. W., Rapoff, M. A., Waldron, S. A., Gragg, R. A., Bernstein, B. H., & Lindsley, C. B. (1996). Chronic pain and emotional distress in children and adolescents. *Developmental and Behavioral Pediatrics, 17*(3), 154–161.

Varni, J. W., Thompson, K. L., & Hanson, V. (1987). The Varni/Thompson pediatric pain questionnaire. Chronic musculoskeletal pain in juvenile arthritis. *Pain, 28*(1), 27–38.

Varni, J. W., & Walco, G. A. (1988). Chronic and recurrent pain associated with pediatric chronic diseases. *Issues in Comprehensive Pediatric Nursing, 11*, 145–158.

Varni, J. W., Waldron, S. A., Gragg, R. A., Rapoff, M. A., Bernstein, B. H., Lindsley, C. B., & Newcomb, M. D. (1996). Development of the Waldon/Varni pediatric pain coping inventory. *Pain, 67*, 141–150.

Walco, G. A., Dampier, C. D., Hartstein, G., Djordjevic, D., & Miller, L. (1990). The relationship between recurrent clinical pain and pain threshold in children. In D. C. Tyler & E. J. Krane (Eds.), *Advances in Pain Research and Therapy: Vol. 15. Pediatric pain* (pp. 333–340). New York: Raven Press.

Walco, G. A., Varni, J. W., & Ilowite, N. T. (1992). Cognitive-behavioral pain management in children with juvenile arthritis. *Pediatrics, 89*(6, Pt. 1), 1075–1079.

Wallace, C. A., & Levinson, J. E. (1991). Juvenile arthritis: Outcome and treatment for the 1990s. *Rheumatoid Disease Clinics of North America, 17*(4), 891–905.

Wallach, J. (1983). *Interpretation of pediatric tests.* Boston, MA: Little, Brown, and Company.

Wright, F. V., Kimber, J. L., Law, M., Goldsmith, C. H., Crombie, V., & Dent, P. (1996). The Juvenile Arthritis Functional Status Index (JASI): A validation study. *Journal of Rheumatology, 23,* 1066–1079.

Zeltzer, L., & LeBaron, S. (1982). Hypnosis and nonhypnotic techniques for the reduction of pain and anxiety during painful procedures in children and adolescents with cancer. *Journal of Pediatrics, 101,* 1032–1035.

CHAPTER 4

Cancer in Children

Ida M. (Ki) Moore

Then are approximately 11,000 new cases of childhood cancer each year in the United States. The incidence is greater in adolescents between the ages of 14–18 years (20 cases per 100,000) than in children younger than 15 years (14 cases per 100,000). Based on current incidence data, cancer develops in approximately 1 in 333 persons in the United States before the age of 20 (Lukens, 1994). The most common pediatric tumors include: leukemia (31.4%), central nervous system (CNS) tumors (17.6%), lymphoma (12.4%), soft tissue sarcomas (7.1%), neuroblastoma (6.6%), Wilms' tumor (6.4%), and bone tumors (5.0%) (Miller, Young, & Novakovic, 1995).

EPIDEMIOLOGY

There has been a modest increase in cancer occurrence over the past 2 decades. An analysis of population-based data from nine registries of the Surveillance, Epidemiology, and End Results (SEER) Program of the National Cancer Institute has demonstrated a 1% average yearly increase in the incidence rates of all malignant neoplasms combined for children 14 years of age or younger (Gurney et al., 1996). Recent data, however, suggest a leveling off or a slight decline in the overall incidence rates (Ries et al., 1999). The increased incidence of childhood cancer does not differ by gender, but is slightly greater for black than for white children, and is most apparent among children less than 3 years of age. Rates for astroglial tumors, rhabdomyosarcoma, germ cell tumors, and osteogenic sarcoma increased 2% or more per year, while neuroblastoma and retinoblastoma in children less than 1 year of age increased 3.1% and 5.4%, respectively (Gurney et al., 1996). Earlier detection, environmental factors, and interactions between genetic traits and environmental exposures have been proposed as plausible explanations for the increasing trends in childhood cancer. Therefore, increased research efforts are being directed toward epidemiologic studies of potential causes and risk factors for individual childhood cancers.

Greater knowledge of tumor biology, improved methods of detection and diagnosis, multimodal therapy, and supportive care interventions to manage the side effects of treatment have resulted in dramatic improvements in long-term disease-free survival, especially for acute lymphoblastic leukemia (ALL), non-Hodgkins' lymphoma, and Wilms' tumor (Cancer Statistics, 1997). Overall 5-year disease-free survival increased from 45% in 1970 to approximately 80% percent in 1995 (Barr, Freedman, & Fryer, 1996). The impressive strides in survival have resulted in a dramatic decline in cancer mortality. For example, of the nearly 60,000 deaths in 1995 among individuals less than 20 years of age, less than 4% (2275) were due to cancer (Ries et al., 1999).

RISK FACTORS FOR CHILDHOOD CANCERS

Associations between prenatal or postnatal environmental (e.g., hydrocarbons, paints, benzene, and pesticides) and drug exposures (e.g., amphetamines, diuretics, and phenytoin) and risk for childhood cancer have only recently been investigated. To date, the findings from reported studies are mostly inconclusive and sometimes controversial. Limitations of most published epidemiologic studies of childhood cancer include use of parental recall rather than a sophisticated exposure assessment, and small sample sizes (Ries et al., 1999; Zahm & Devesa, 1995). Furthermore, the short latency period between conception and early age of occurrence for most pediatric tumors narrows the window of time for investigating the carcinogenic effects of environmental exposures.

There is modest evidence that maternal diet and alcohol or other drug consumption during the index pregnancy are either protective against or associated with an increased risk for some pediatric cancers. A case control study of 166 children diagnosed with primitive neuroectodermal tumors (PNET) of the brain (median age at diagnosis was 33 months) was conducted using random digit telephone dialing. Controls were matched for age and race; telephone interviews with mothers included questions on the frequency of consumption of alcohol, vitamin and mineral supplements, and 53 foods during pregnancy (Bunin et al., 1993). Univariate analyses demonstrated a significant protective effect for multivitamin use during the first 6 weeks after the last menstrual period (odds ratio [OR] = 0.56, p = 0.02), and for iron (OR = 0.43, p = 0.004), calcium (OR = 0.42, p = 0.05), and vitamin C (OR = 0.35, p = 0.04) supplements. The consumption of fruits and vegetables conferred large reductions in risk for those in the highest quartile of food intake group (OR = 0.28 to 0.37, respectively, p ≤ 0.05). The protective effects of folate, early multivitamin use, and iron supplements were also supported by multivariate analyses. The protective effects of folate against PNET were thought to parallel the protective effects against neural tube defects. The neural tube is formed and closed during the first 4 weeks of gestation (6 weeks after the last menstrual period), and the neuroepithelial cells that line the neural tube are the precursor cells of PNETs (Bunin et al., 1993).

Maternal alcohol consumption during the index pregnancy, especially during the second and third trimesters has been associated with an increased risk for acute leukemia. A case control study of parents of children diagnosed with leukemia at 18 months of age or younger involved telephone interviews (Shu et al., 1996). Mothers were asked questions about events and exposures prior to and during the index pregnancy and birth, occupational, reproductive, and family medical history. Forty percent of mothers of case patients reported ever drinking during the pregnancy as compared to 31% of the mothers of control subjects. Using the group of mothers who never drank during the month prior to and during pregnancy as the referent, maternal drinking during the second and/or third trimester was associated with a 2.28-fold elevated risk for ALL and a 10.48 elevated risk for acute myelocytic leukemia (AML). The risk of AML was positively associated with the total amount of alcohol consumed during the index pregnancy. Infants of mothers who consumed more than 20 drinks had a 3.13-fold higher risk of AML than did infants who had no in utero alcohol exposure.

Maternal cigarette smoking was not associated with an increased risk of childhood leukemia (Shu et al., 1996), however, an 11-fold increased risk of AML has been associated with maternal use of mind-altering drugs (primarily marijuana) just prior to the index pregnancy, and parents' use of cocaine and marijuana significantly increased the risk of rhabdomyosarcoma (Robison, Buckley, & Bunin, 1995). Maternal prenatal exposure to diuretics for hypertension, tranquilizers, and nonprescription pain relievers have been associated with an increased risk of neuroblastoma, a tumor of sympathetic nervous system origin (Schwartzbaum, 1992; Kramer et al., 1987).

History of maternal fetal loss (spontaneous abortion or miscarriage) has also been investigated as a risk factor for childhood ALL (Yeazel et al., 1995). A case control study using a Children's Cancer Group database compared 1,753 children with acute leukemia with 839 community control subjects and 2081 nonleukemia cancer control subjects. History of any previous fetal loss, number of previous fetal losses, and antecedent fetal loss in the mother's entire reproductive history were significant risk factors for the development of ALL in the 0–2 and the 2–4 year age groups. The risk was greatest for children diagnosed with ALL between the ages of 0–2 years. In this young age group, history of any previous fetal loss was associated with a relative risk (RR) of 4.94, and two or more fetal losses was associated with a RR of 24.76. The risk for ALL increased significantly with an increasing number of fetal losses in the entire reproductive history (p < 0.001). Hypothesized explanations include genetic factors predisposing to an early onset of ALL, and parental exposures to environmental agents that not only increase the risk of fetal loss, but may also result in childhood ALL (Yeazel et al., 1995).

Some parental occupational exposures (e.g., carpenter, mechanic, painter, dryer, and machinist) have also been associated with an increased risk of childhood cancer. Feingold, Savitz, and John (1992) used a job exposure matrix to assign parental exposures for at least 6 months during the year prior to the birth of the index child in a case control study of parents of 252 children with cancer and 222 controls selected by random digit dialing. Paternal exposure to creosote, polysiloxanes, and vanadium had adjusted odds ratios (OR) of 2.0 or greater for any childhood cancer. Paternal exposure to aniline and anthracene were associated with an increased risk for ALL (OR ≥ 2.0); exposure to creosote and beryllium was associated with an increased risk of brain tumors (OR = 3.7 and 2.1, respectively). Many mothers did not work outside the home, resulting in fewer exposures. Maternal exposures to benzene, petroleum/coke pitch/tar and soot, however, were associated with elevated OR (1.9–3.3) in relation to total cancers.

Bunin and others (1990) reported that paternal occupations in the metal industry or in the military were associated with sporadic heritable retinoblastoma and that employment as welders or machinists before and after conception was associated with the nonheritable form of the disease (OR = 4.0 and 5.0, respectively). The sporadic heritable form of retinoblastoma is thought to result from new germinal mutations, therefore, preconception exposures of the father but not the mother are more likely to be linked to disease. In the nonheritable form of retinoblastoma, however, postconception exposures are also important. An intriguing finding is that significantly more cases than controls in the nonheritable group had maternal grandfathers who were farmers (OR = 10.0). One possible explanation is that women whose fathers were farmers would have been exposed to pesticides while growing up on a farm (Bunin et al., 1990). Some pesticides can be stored for extended periods of time in human fat, resulting in a higher body burden of pesticides that could adversely affect the fetus after conception.

Paternal exposure to low level radiation has also been associated with an increased risk of infant leukemia. Telephone interviews were conducted with mothers and fathers (when available) of cases (n = 302) and controls (n = 558). Detailed information on parental preconception diagnostic X-ray exposure and in utero radiation exposure was collected. Risk of leukemia was significantly increased among children whose fathers reported ever having preconception X-ray exposure (Shu et al., 1994). The risk of ALL increased with the number of X rays the father received to the upper gastrointestinal (GI), lower GI and lower abdomen, and chest. The highest risk for ALL was related to two or more X rays of the lower GI tract and lower abdomen (OR = 3.78). Higher risks were also linked to exposures closer to conception. The number of mothers exposed to low levels of radiation was small, however, X-ray exposure in the month prior to conception of the index child was related to an increased risk (OR = 4.5) of infant leukemia. The possibility of recall bias among parents of children with cancer was acknowledged, however, differences between maternal and paternal exposures and the pattern of exposures reported minimized the potential threat of recall bias. The findings could not be attributed to differences in underlying diseases that required X-ray examinations or medications that might result in germ cell mutations. The link between preconception X-ray exposure and infant ALL indicate a potential role for germline transmission of mutation or genomic instability in the development of cancer in young children (Shu et al., 1994.) As noted by the investigators, direct evidence linking genetic markers to preconception exposures are essential for resolving the current controversy about germline transmission of leukemia.

Children may also be directly exposed to carcinogens that increase their risk for cancer. One of the limitations in identifying environmental risks is the short latency period between the time of exposure and the early age at the time of occurrence of most pediatric tumors. Leiss and Savitz (1995) conducted a case control study of 252 children diagnosed with cancer in the Denver area between 1976 and 1983, and 222 control subjects matched by age, sex, and geographic location. Exposure data were collected through parental interviews about dates of occupancy, extermination for insects or pests, yard treatment with insecticides or herbicides, and use of hanging pest strips for insect control. The most striking findings include a strong association between yard treatment and soft tissue sarcomas (OR = 3.9 to 4.1), and between the use of pest strips and childhood tumors, especially leukemia (OR = 1.7 to 3.0).

The other environmental exposure that has been explored as possibly linked to cancer in children is electromagnetic fields. There is limited evidence for an association between elevated risk of ALL and level of exposure to electromagnetic fields (Feychting et al., 1995). Others have reported a small to no risk for ALL or brain tumors after exposure to electromagnetic fields (Ries et al., 1999). Overall, there is limited information about the relevant exposure measure, the biological mechanism(s) by which exposure to magnetic fields are carcinogenic, and relevant health outcomes.

EARLY DETECTION AND SCREENING

Currently, there are almost no effective early detection and screening methods for pediatric malignancies. Lack of screening methods is due to the early age of onset for most tumors, and the lack of sensitive markers for early detection. Mass screening of infants for neuroblastoma, a tumor of sympathetic nervous system tissue origin, was done in Japan. The screening involved measuring vanillymandelic acid (VMA) and homovanillic acid (HVA) levels in urine. Urinary VMA and HVA are frequently elevated in neuroblastoma because they are metabolites of catecholamines. The incidence of advanced disease did not increase either before or after initiation of the screening program. Furthermore, the majority of cases of neuroblastoma detected by mass screening were in an early stage, demonstrated favorable prognostic factors, and did not require aggressive therapy (Suita et al., 1996). Many of these cases of neuroblastoma may have eventually spontaneously regressed (which can occur in infancy) or have been clinically detected with a good prognosis. Because of these and similar findings, mass screening programs have not been widely implemented, and are of questionable benefit.

DISEASE PROCESSES

The majority of pediatric cancers arise from the mesodermal germ layer, which normally differentiates into connective tissue, bone, cartilage, muscle, blood and blood vessels, kidney, lymphatic and lymphoid organs. Central nervous system tumors arise from neuroectodermal tissue (Mooney, 1993).

Malignant transformation is a multistage process involving initiation, promotion, progression, and metastasis. Each stage involves one or more genetic alterations that disrupt the regulatory balance between cellular differentiation and proliferation (Malkin & Portwine, 1994). The genetic alterations may be inherited or sporadic, and interact with, as yet, poorly understood environmental factors (Mott, 1995; Rubinitz & Crist, 1997).

Initiation (damage to DNA) involves the inappropriate activation of proto-oncogenes (normal growth promoting genes) to oncogenes (genes that encode for aberrant cellular growth and proliferation), or the inactivation or deletion of suppressor genes that normally inhibit cellular proliferation. Promotion is the second event in carcinogenesis that stimulates transformed cells to proliferate. Progression refers to tumor invasion of surrounding tissue and involves the accumulation of additional genetic alterations. Metastasis, the final stage of carcinogenesis, involves the spread of cancer cells to distant sites and is often accompanied by development of drug resistance. Metastatic tumors are usually genetically diverse (multiclonal) and drug resistant.

The two broad categories of genes involved in the development of pediatric cancers are *dominant* oncogenes and *recessive* suppressor genes. Proto-oncogenes encode signals for regulatory proteins for cell growth and proliferation. Translocation and gene fusion events are the most common mechanisms of inappropriate activation from a proto-oncogene to an oncogene.

Other less common mechanisms involved in pediatric tumors include viral insertion, point mutation, and gene amplification (Rubinitz & Crist, 1997). Oncogenes behave in a dominant Mendelian pattern, which means that mutation of only one of the two proto-oncogene alleles is necessary for oncogenesis. Oncogenes can promote cell transformation in several different ways. For example, in B cell leukemia and Burketts' lymphoma, the MYC oncogene encodes for a group of nuclear phosphoproteins that maintain an expanded population of B cell progenitors in a proliferative state, making them more susceptible to further genetic alterations (Mott, 1995).

Suppressor genes encode for proteins that suppress cell growth. Therefore, deletion or inactivation of a tumor suppressor gene contributes to tumor development by removing key constraints on cell proliferation. Retinoblastoma, a rare tumor of the eye, arises as a result of the functional inactivation of the retinoblastoma susceptibility gene (RB1) on the long arm of chromosome 13. The normal gene encodes for a protein that when hypophosphorylated, acts early in the G1 phase of the cell cycle to inhibit proliferation (Mott, 1995). Abnormalities of both copies of RB1 are involved in both the hereditary and nonhereditary forms of retinoblastoma. Children who inherit a germline mutation are also at increased risk for other primary tumors, especially osteosarcoma (Draper, Sanders, & Kinston, 1986). Mutations or deletions of suppressor genes have also been identified for other pediatric malignancies, including Wilms' tumor, sarcomas, brain tumors including PNET, and leukemias (Rubinitz & Crist, 1997).

RECENT ADVANCES IN DISEASE ASSESSMENT AND MANAGEMENT

Assessment of Disease Status

The ability to define tumors by biological characteristics such as cell surface antigens, genetic alterations, and histology is one of the most important recent advances in assessment. Biological characteristics of the tumor are used in combination with other parameters, such as the age of the child, tumor location and degree of spread, presence of metastatic disease, and when appropriate, elevated serum levels of specific markers to determine tumor stage, prognosis, and treatment plan. For example, amplification of the N-MYC oncogene in neuroblastoma is associated with aggressive tumors and a poor treatment outcome, regardless of age or disease stage (Rubinitz & Crist, 1997). Neuroblastoma patients positive for a mutation of the p53 suppressor gene also have a significantly worse prognosis (Layfield et al., 1995). On the other hand, children less than 12 months of age whose tumors do not have N-MYC amplification or p53 mutations, have a much better prognosis than children 2 years of age or older.

For ALL, the specific type of lymphoid cell involved (B or T cell), and the degree of differentiation are important. Leukemia that is classified as early pre-B cell is associated with a more favorable prognosis than either B cell or T cell leukemia. In B-lineage ALL, hyperdiploidy (modal chromosome number greater than 50), and trisomy of chromosomes 4 and 10 are associated with a very good outcome (Martin et al., 1996; Trueworthy, Shuster, & Look, 1992). Translocation between chromosomes 1 and 19 [t (1;19)] is predictive of a less favorable outcome, however, use of more intensive chemotherapy for children with t (1;19) has increased survival from 50% to 80% (Rivera et al., 1991).

Disease Management

The use of aggressive multidrug chemotherapy regimens, often in combination with radiation and surgery has resulted in significant improvements in long-term survival. Autologous and allogenic bone marrow transplant have now become conventional therapy for tumors that previously were considered terminal, such as AML, relapsed or high risk ALL, and advanced stage neuroblastoma. Effective treatment of drug resistant and highly aggressive tumors, however, continues to be a challenge. In order to overcome this challenge, investigators are evaluating the maximum tolerated dose, dose-limiting toxicities, and antitumor activity of new drugs in Phase I and Phase II trials. For example, Paclitaxel, an antimicrotubule agent that disrupts micro-tubule structure and function, has been evaluated for refractory leukemia and solid tumors (Seibel & Reaman, 1996).

The use of a new generation of folate analogs that circumvent resistance to methotrexate (MTX) is another new development in the treatment of childhood cancer. MTX is an antifolate agent that blocks the formation of folic acid, which is essential for maintaining cellular functions, and is very effective in the treatment of childhood ALL. Tumor cells, however, can develop MTX resistance at a number of different reactions in the folate pathway. New antifolate compounds are being tested for unique and poten-tially more potent mechanisms of action in order to improve treatment out-comes and overcome MTX resistance (Hum & Kamen, 1996).

Gene therapy, defined as the insertion of exogenous genetic material into somatic cells with therapeutic intent, is the most recent innovation in the assessment and treatment of childhood cancers (Benaim & Sorrentino, 1996). One application of gene therapy is inserting marker genes into bone marrow cells prior to autologous transplantation. These marker genes have been identified in tumor cells of patients who subsequently relapsed. These findings have documented the importance of *in vitro* tumoricidal purging methods for eradicating residual malignant cells from grafts prior to transplant (Benaim & Sorrentino, 1996). Clinical trials involving gene therapy in pediatric oncology have been approved for implementation. These trials involve insertion of genes that encode for tumoricidal proteins into lymphocytes that bind to tumors, and insertion of suicide genes that convert prodrugs into toxic metabo-lites into tumor cells. These studies offer new, and potentially more effective ways for irradiating tumor cells.

Management of Disease and Treatment-Related Symptoms

Advances in the management of disease and treatment-related symptoms are also important. Growth factors, such as granulocyte macrophage colony stimulating factor (GM-CSF), hasten the recovery of bone marrow progenitor cells from the suppressive effects of chemotherapy, which decreases the risk for sepsis. A new class of antiemetic drugs, serotonin antagonists, selectively blocks serotonin (5-HT$_3$) receptors of the gut and visceral afferent nerves. These drugs, used in combination with other agents such as dexamethasone, are particularly effective in decreasing the nausea and vomiting associated with many chemotherapy regimens (Ettinger, 1995). These pharmacologic advances have decreased the morbidity associated with aggressive cancer treatment.

Behavioral coping strategies are also important for managing chemotherapy-induced nausea and vomiting. The KIDCOPE, an inventory designed to assess cognitive and behavioral coping strategies used by children between the ages of 6–18 years, was modified to investigate chemotherapy-induced nausea and vomiting symptoms in 57 patients undergoing active treatment for cancers other than central nervous system tumors. The distress associated with nausea and vomiting was reported as somewhat to very much by 32% and 47% of the subjects, respectively (Tyc et al., 1995a). The most frequently used coping strategies for nausea included wishful thinking, emotional regulation, distraction, and social support. Emotional regulation and wishful thinking were primarily used to manage emesis. The median number of coping strategies used by subjects was seven. Coping strategies were more effective for managing symptoms related to nausea than to emesis. The group of subjects who were rated as Successful Coper reported minimal symptom distress and perceived their coping strategies as highly effective. They tended to receive less emetogenic chemotherapy and tended to use problem solving and social support for coping with nausea. The findings suggest that patients who continue to use ineffective strategies and experience increasing distress should be targeted for interventions designed to teach more effective coping behaviors (Tyc et al., 1995a).

Nutritional problems are also a common concern for pediatric cancer patients because malnutrition has been associated with decreased tolerance of chemotherapy, increased incidence of infection, and a worse prognosis. Weight loss and malnutrition occur in approximately one third of pediatric cancer patients, and the percentage is higher among those with advanced disease. Decreased appetite, increased metabolic rate, taste changes, nausea and vomiting, and behavioral/environmental factors, such as learned food aversions, are common problems that contribute to poor oral intake and malnutrition. Tyc and colleagues (1995b) investigated which nutritional and treatment-related variables discriminated between patients who were and were not referred for nutritional intervention. A significantly higher percentage of patients in the referred group had received prior radiation therapy, had poor oral intake and mucositis/stomatitis in the month prior to referral than those in the nonreferred group (X^2 = 9.0 to 116.03, p ≤ 0.003). Poor oral intake in the 30 days preceding referral was the best overall predictor of need for nutritional support (Tyc et al., 1995b). The investigators suggest that preventive behavioral interventions and nutritional counseling designed to increase caloric intake over time may offer relatively noninvasive and cost effective methods for management of nutritional problems in pediatric oncology patients.

Serum levels of antioxidant vitamins, beta-carotene, zinc, selenium, and cholesterol, and related proteins were measured in two reported studies of newly diagnosed pediatric oncology patients and cancer-free controls (Malvy et al., 1997; Malvy et al., 1993). In general, the mean serum concentrations of retinol, beta-carotene, zinc, alpha-tocopherol, and cholesterol were lower in cancer cases than in controls, however, there were some differences in micronutrient deficiencies by tumor type. The causes for the findings were thought to be multifactorial, including increased cellular demand, altered biosynthesis in the liver, high receptor-mediated uptake and degradation by some malignant cells, generation of oxygen-free radicals by radiation, some anticancer drugs, activated granulocytes, and insufficient intake. The results suggest that preventive nutritional interventions need to be individualized to meet specific needs and that supplementation with antioxidants, even at higher levels than that administered in enteral or parenteral nutrition, could be required in patients undergoing highly toxic cancer treatment (Malvy et al., 1997). The addition of micronutrients, such as glutamine, arginine, and omega-3 fatty acids to enteral feedings has also been proposed to have a positive effect on the nutritional status of children receiving intensive chemotherapy at a significantly lower cost than total parental nutrition (Ford, Whitlock, & Pietsch, 1997).

Recent research has identified fatigue as an important symptom experienced by children and adolescents with cancer. Hockenberry-Eaton and colleagues (1998) conducted focus groups in order to define and describe fatigue experienced by children and adolescents with cancer (n = 29 participants between the ages of 7–16). Children described both physical and mental symptoms, such as weakness and being tired, feeling upset, and not being able to participate in sports. Adolescents also described both physical and mental fatigue. Examples of adolescent descriptions of fatigue include causing changes in their body, feeling sorry for self, physical symptoms such as dizziness, nausea, hot and cold flashes, and falling asleep anywhere. Future studies will involve the development of instruments to measure fatigue and the evaluation of specific interventions to alleviate this often overlooked symptom experienced by pediatric oncology patients.

Frequent hospitalizations resulting in time away from school and peers, painful invasive procedures, and treatment-related physical changes, such as alopecia, are common psychosocial stressors experienced by pediatric oncology patients. Hockenberry-Eaton and others (1994) investigated relationships between acute and chronic cancer stressors, protective factors, and the physiological and psychological responses to stressors experienced during treatment for childhood cancer. Acute stressors included intermittent episodes, which may be frightening or painful over a short period of time (e.g., bone marrow aspirates, lumbar punctures, or intravenous chemotherapy), while chronic stressors were the day-to-day experiences of living with cancer. Protective factors were defined as child, family, and environmental attributes that alter the perception of cancer. The sample was comprised of 48 children with cancer receiving chemotherapy; data were collected during two outpatient clinic visits. Mean epinephrine levels, a physiologic measure of acute stress, was elevated above normal levels during both clinic visits. Family expressiveness and global self-worth accounted for 20% of the variance in epinephrine levels during the second clinic visit. The mean norepinephrine levels were elevated, but within the normal range for age. Perceived support from friends accounted for 12% of the variance in norepinephrine level. Two other independent variables, family activities and recreation and family cultural orientation, explained 32% of the variance in state anxiety.

Varni and others (1994a) also documented the importance of perceived support for coping with cancer. Their study involved 30 children between the ages of 8–13 years with newly diagnosed cancer. Perceived classmate social support significantly predicted depressive symptoms, state anxiety, trait anxiety, social anxiety, and behavior problems (Varni et al., 1994a). Perceived social support from teachers predicted externalizing behavior problems, such as acting out and aggression. The investigators hypothesized that social skills training may assist the child with cancer in overcoming the disruptions of normal social development through enhancing social competence.

Greater knowledge about stressors and protective factors that influence coping with and adjustment to a life-threatening illness such as cancer is important. For example, Hinds (1988) reported that hopefulness is an important factor for adolescents experiencing life-threatening illness, and that adolescents with cancer had hope for others as well as for self.

ADVANCES IN LONG-TERM SURVIVAL AND MANAGEMENT OF LATE EFFECTS

Five-year relative survival from childhood cancer has increased from 56% between 1974–1976 to 75% between 1989–1995; for childhood ALL, the most common pediatric tumor, survival rates increased from 53% to 81% during the same time interval (Greenlee et al., 2000). It is predicted that by 2010, 1 in 250 individuals between the ages of 15–45 will be a long-term survivor of childhood cancer. Using an average age of 5 years at the time of cancer diagnosis, and 77 years as the projected length of life, approximately 72 years of every childhood cancer survivor's life is influenced by the late effects of the disease and treatment. According to Bleyer (1990), the dramatic improvement in survival is worthwhile only if the quality of survival justifies the increased prolongation of life. There is a growing body of knowledge about the late effects of childhood cancer and its treatment and the impact of these late effects on quality of life.

In contrast to the acute side effects of treatment which are caused by the effects of radiation and chemotherapy on proliferative cells, late effects become observable months to years after the completion of treatment, may be due to different mechanisms of injury, and can range in severity from mild to life threatening. Late effects have been identified as affecting almost every organ system. The risk for a particular late effect is dependent upon the type and total dose of chemotherapy or radiation received, the developmental stage of the organ at the time of treatment, and sometimes, gender.

The psychological consequences of surviving a life-threatening illness have also been described; the risk for these emotional late effects is influenced by age at the time of cancer treatment, type of treatment received and any residual effects of the treatment, and the amount and type of support received by peers and family.

Cognitive and psychological late effects are discussed below. Issues related to quality of life for long-term survivors of childhood cancer are also addressed. For more detailed and comprehensive information on the assessment and management of late effects, the reader is referred to *Survivors of Childhood Cancer: Assessment and Management* (Schwartz et al., 1994).

Cognitive Late Effects

Treatment of the central nervous system (CNS) with radiation and chemotherapy can result in cognitive impairments, including declines in general intelligence and academic achievement scores as well as deficits in visual spatial, verbal fluency, memory, and speed of information processing. There is some evidence that higher doses of radiation (≥ 24 Gray [Gy]) are associated with more serious late effects. Several investigators (Butler et al., 1994; Jankovic et al., 1994; Moore et al., 1991; Mulhern, Fairclough, & Ochs, 1991), however, have found that children with ALL treated with 18 Gy also experience a spectrum of cognitive impairments. There is increasing evidence that systemic treatment with high doses of drugs, such as MTX, that cross the blood brain barrier, and intrathecal chemotherapy, can also result in impairments that are serious enough to affect school performance adversely (Butler et al., 1994; Kaufmann et al., 1996; Mulhern, Fairclough, & Ochs, 1991; Mulhern et al., 1988; Ochs et al., 1991). Espy and colleagues (2000) used growth curve analysis to examine neuropsychological outcome and treatment-related change in 30 children who had received either intrathecal MTX or triple intrathecal chemotherapy plus intermediate dose systemic MTX. Modest declines in specific areas of neuropsychological function, such as arithmetic, visual motor integration, and verbal fluency, were observed. In addition, children who received both intrathecal and systemic chemotherapy for CNS treatment had poorer visual motor integration 4 years after treatment and a faster rate of decline in visual motor integration skills (Espy et al., 2000).

The mechanisms of injury to the CNS following radiation and chemotherapy are not completely understood, however, documented increases in the concentration of cerebral spinal fluid phospholipids suggest damage to cell membranes that can initiate inflammation, ischemia, or apoptosis (Mollova et al., 1995; Moore, 1995; Moore et al., 2000). Recently, Moore and others (2000) observed that increased concentrations of specific phospholipids in cerebral spinal fluid of children receiving CNS treatment for ALL were negatively correlated with cognitive and academic abilities.

Computed tomography (CT) examinations of 196 children during (n = 125) and/or after (n = 71) treatment with ALL involved measurements of the width of the subarachnoid compartments (Prassopoulos et al., 1996). Dilatation of the CSF spaces, indicative of diffuse brain atrophy was observed in CT evaluations performed during (74%) and after (65%) cessation of treatment. The highest incidence of brain atrophy (78%) occurred during the administration of chemotherapy, but all children younger than 2 years of age at the time of treatment exhibited atrophy. The study did not include measures of cognitive function (Prassopoulos et al., 1996); thus, the potential relationship between brain atrophy and cognitive impairments is unknown.

Children who receive CNS therapy are at risk for school-related and emotional problems. Sawyer and colleagues (1988) investigated the prevalence of emotional and behavioral problems in a group of 32 children and adolescents treated for leukemia (mean age = 13.4 years, SD = 2.9) compared to siblings (mean age = 12.5 years, SD = 2.3) and a matched control group (mean age = 13.5 years, SD = 2.9) from the general population. School performance of the leukemia group was significantly below that of the comparison groups. Overall learning and total adaptive functioning were two behaviors noted by teachers to be especially problematic. Results from a large retrospective cohort study of 593 survivors of childhood ALL and 409 sibling controls demonstrated that the ALL survivors were significantly more likely than their sibling controls to enter a special education or learning disabled program (p < .01) (Haupt et al., 1994). There are no reports of large-scale intervention studies designed to improve academic outcomes of children receiving CNS treatment. Moore and colleagues (2000), however, recently demonstrated a significant improvement (p ≤ 0.01) in academic arithmetic abilities in a small group (n = 8) of children who had treatment-related academic problems after 40–50 hrs of a skill-building tutorial intervention. Similar gains in academic abilities were not observed in a comparison group (n = 7) who did not receive the intervention.

Psychological Late Effects

The experiences of completing cancer therapy from the perspective of the child and adolescent were the focus of a qualitative study by Haase and Rostad (1994). Six themes were derived from open-ended interviews with seven participants between the ages of 5–18 years who had completed cancer therapy during the past year and who remained in remission. The six theme categories were: (1) a gradual realization of completion, (2) hierarchical and cyclical recurrence fears, (3) completion embedded within the cancer experience, (4) seeking a new normal, (5) modifying relationships, and (6) resolution and moving on. The formulated meanings and theme clusters revealed the positive and negative aspects of completing cancer treatment.

Mulhern and colleagues (1989) observed a significantly higher incidence of deficiencies in social competence and an increased frequency of behavioral problems among cancer survivors compared to general population norms on the Child Behavior Checklist. The most frequent observed problems included poor school performance and somatic complaints. Sixty-seven percent of the sample displayed one or more abnormalities on the Child Behavior Checklist, which is significantly greater (p < 0.005) than in the general population. Older age at the time of the evaluation, treatment with whole brain radiation, and residence in a single-parent household were associated with an increased risk for psychological problems (Mulhern et al., 1989).

Other researchers have also documented psychosocial adjustment problems among long-term survivors. Varni and colleagues (1994b) investigated psychological adjustment correlates of perceived stress in a sample of 39 participants between the ages of 13–23 years (mean age = 17.4 years). Psychological distress was measured by the Symptom Checklist 90-Revised (SCL-90), and general self-esteem was measured by the Self-Perception Profile for Adolescents. Older age was moderately correlated with a greater intensity of symptoms in the areas of depression, anxiety, interpersonal sensitivity, somatization, and obsessive-compulsiveness (measured by SCL-90 subscales, ($r = .27$ to $.41$, $p < 0.05$ to < 0.005), and the diagnosis of leukemia was moderately correlated with greater intensity of symptoms related to psychotism and paranoid ideation ($r = .28$ to $.31$, $p < 0.05$). Higher perceived stress significantly predicted 24% of the variance in the Global Severity Index from the SCL-90 ($p < 0.001$), and 13 to 24% of the variance in 12 measures of adjustment, including depression, anxiety, interpersonal sensitivity, obsessive-compulsiveness, and general self-esteem ($p < 0.05$ to < 0.0001) (Varni et al., 1994).

Sloper, Larcombe, and Charlton (1994) described psychosocial adjustment of 5-year survivors of childhood cancer compared with a group of healthy school peers. Cancer survivors had significantly higher scores on parent- and teacher-rated scales of behavioral problems, and significantly lower scores on teacher ratings of concentration, academic progress, and popularity with peers ($p < 0.05$). Cancer survivors were more likely to have behavioral problems if their parents' levels of active, problem-focused coping were low and the parents had high levels of a passive focused strategy referred to as wishful thinking. Varni and colleagues (1994a) pointed out the need for identifying risk and protective factors for psychological adjustment, and for the development of behavioral interventions to modify or increase stress management strategies.

Mackie and colleagues (2000) also reported higher rates of psychosocial problems among childhood cancer survivors. A sample of 102 survivors of childhood leukemia or Wilms' tumor and 102 unrelated healthy controls completed standardized measures of interpersonal and social-role performance and intellectual ability to assess past and current functioning. Mean scores were significantly higher (indicating poorer functioning) in the domains of love/sex relationships, friendship, nonspecific social contacts, and day-to-day functioning. Problems in close relationships were associated with more recent cancer treatment and poorer coping was associated with lower intelligence. The investigators proposed that a more recent disruption of social relationships could explain the relationship between close relationships and recent treatment, while the relationship between intellectual abilities and coping could be a direct effect of treatment-related cognitive impairments.

Although the majority of studies of long-term cancer survivors have focused on children with leukemia or Wilms' tumor, Kornblith and colleagues (1998) reported that survivors of advanced stage Hodgkin's disease were at greater risk for high psychological distress scores than were survivors of acute leukemia. Two hundred and seventy-three Hodgkin's disease survivors and 206 adult leukemia survivors were interviewed by telephone about their psychological adjustment and problems they attributed to having been treated for cancer. Hodgkin's disease survivors reported significantly greater psychological distress, poorer sexual functioning, greater fatigue, and greater conditioned nausea than did leukemia survivors. The overall prevalence rate of high distress among leukemia survivors was 14% greater than the expected rate in the general population; however, the overall prevalence rate of high distress among survivors of Hodgkin's disease was 21% (3 times the expected rate in the general population).

The length of time since the cancer diagnosis can have a negative influence on some of these psychosocial outcomes. In a study of 48 children with cancer receiving treatment in an outpatient setting, Hockenberry-Eaton, Dilorio, and Kemp (1995) found that the number of months since the diagnosis correlated negatively with the children's perception of global self-worth and athletic competence. The correlation was greater for patients who had experienced a relapse than for those who had not. Trait anxiety was also higher among relapsed patients. Children with lower self-perception and higher trait anxiety scores reported experiencing more cancer-related stressors. An interesting finding that has also been reported by others was that children with leukemia reported higher levels of chronic cancer stressors than those with solid tumors. As noted by the investigators, this finding may be related to the 2.5–3 years of unrelenting treatment for ALL, in comparison to therapy for solid tumors that can range from 6 months to 2 years (Hockenberry-Eaton, Dilorio, & Kemp, 1995).

Decision making, risk behaviors, and health practices can also be influenced by a previous cancer experience. Hollen and Hobbie (1996) compared decision-making quality and prevalence of risk-taking behaviors, including smoking, alcohol, and illicit drug use of 52 cancer-surviving adolescents with that of their peers. The investigators used a Decision Making Quality Scale that assesses the degree to which a person adheres to seven quality decision-making criteria during consequential decision making. The majority of peers adhered to only three and the cancer survivors to only two of the seven quality decision-making criteria, suggesting that both groups lacked effective decision-making skills. There were fewer risk behaviors reported by teen survivors in comparison to their most influential peers, however, cigarette smoking and alcohol use of the teen survivors was comparable with the general population. This finding is in contrast to a survey of 40 long-term cancer survivors in which the reported prevalence of alcohol and tobacco use was < 10% among respondents < 18 years of age (Mulhern et al., 1995). Despite the high percentage of participants and their parents who believed it was important to protect the survivor's health (60% and 83.6%, respectively), 25% of the sample reported brushing their teeth once a day or less frequently, infrequently eating balanced meals, and infrequently wearing seat belts. Investigators stress the need to increase the scope of long-term follow-up care to include health risk and health protecting behaviors that may reduce or minimize the late sequelae of treatment and improve life quality (Mulhern et al., 1995).

Quality of life issues for pediatric oncology patients have become increasing important. The following definition of quality of life was put forth by participants in an American Cancer Society Workshop on Quality of Life in Children's Cancer:

> Quality of life (QOL) in pediatric oncology is multidimensional. It includes but is not limited to, the social, physical, and emotional functioning of the child and adolescent, and when indicated, his/her family. Measurement of QOL must be from the perspective of the child, adolescent, and family, and it must be sensitive to the changes that occur throughout development. (Bradlyn et al., 1996, 1333–1334)

An increasing number of clinical trials comparing alternative therapies for pediatric tumors are including QOL endpoints to compare treatment-related toxicities, evaluate prognostic factors, such as performance status at the time of randomization to treatment regimen, describe the late effects or survivorship issues, and to identify problems for which interventions may be appropriate (Bradlyn et al., 1996; Bradlyn & Pollack, 1996). Measurement of quality of life in children and adolescents with cancer has been limited by the availability of developmentally appropriate instruments that measure cancer specific concerns, are responsive to change over time, and have sound psychometric properties.

FUTURE DIRECTIONS FOR BIOBEHAVIORAL RESEARCH AND PRACTICE IN PEDIATRIC ONCOLOGY

Knowledge about the biological and genetic factors involved in carcinogenesis has increased dramatically over the past decade; this knowledge has contributed to improved and more sophisticated methods for assessment and staging of tumors. There have also been advances in the successful treatment of many pediatric cancers, such that long-term disease free survival approaches 80%, however, effective treatment of tumors with some specific genetic characteristics or that have become drug resistant remain a significant challenge. Information about acute and late toxicities has come from increasing interest and concern about the effects of aggressive treatment modalities on the child's and adolescent's current and future life quality.

There are a limited number of investigations that interface the biological and behavioral dimensions of the illness experience. There are even fewer studies that have systematically evaluated the efficacy of interdisciplinary interventions designed to prevent or remediate treatment-related sequelae such as lower self-esteem, decreased social competence, depression, and cognitive impairments.

Jan van Eyes, a well-known pediatric oncologist, eloquently described the "truly cured child." *Biological* cure means that the disease is not discernable by any objective measure, and that the individual dies in old age from unrelated causes. *Psychological* cure means that the child is at ease with having or having had cancer, and past and current events are incorporated into his or her total experienced reality. *Social* cure requires that the child is accepted in society as if the disease were a relatively irrelevant incident. According to van Eyes (1991), "the way we care for the child determines the cure; the cure should not determine the care." Achieving the goal of the truly cured child will require a multidisciplinary approach to the development of interventions that successfully meet the biobehavioral challenges of childhood cancer.

REFERENCES

Barr, R., Freedman, M., & Fryer, C. (1996). Challenges in childhood cancer and blood diseases. *Journal of Pediatric Hematology/Oncology, 18*(1), 3–9.

Benaim, E., & Sorrentino, B. P. (1996). Gene therapy in pediatric oncology. *Investigational New Drugs, 14*, 87–99.

Bleyer, A. (1990). The impact of childhood cancer on the United States and the world. *CA: A Cancer Journal for Clinicians, 40*, 355–367.

Bleyer, W. A. (1995). The past and future of cancer in the young. *Pediatric Dentistry, 17*(4), 285–290.

Bradlyn, A. S., & Pollock, B. H. (1996). Quality of life research in the pediatric oncology group: 1991–1995. *Journal of the National Cancer Institute Monographs, 20*, 49–53.

Bradlyn, A. S., Ritchey, A. K., Harris, C. V., Moore, I. M., O'Brien, R. T., Parson, S. K., Patterson, K., & Pollock, B. H. (1996). Quality of life research in pediatric oncology. *Cancer, 78*(6), 1333–1339.

Bunin, G. R., Kuijten, R. R., Buckley, J. D., Rorke, L. B., & Meadows, A. (1993). Relation between maternal diet and subsequent primitive neuroectodermal brain tumors in young children. *The New England Journal of Medicine, 329*(8), 536–541.

Bunin, G. R., Petrakova, A., Meadows, A. T., Emanuel, B. S., Buckley, J. D., Woods, W. G., & Hammond, G. D. (1990). Occupations of parents of children with retinoblastoma: A report from the children's cancer study group. *Cancer Research, 50*, 7129–7133.

Butler, R. W., Hill, J. M., Steinherz, P. G., Meyers, P. A., & Finlay, J. L. (1994). Neuropsychologic effects of cranial irradiation, intrathecal methotrexate, and systemic methotrexate in childhood cancer. *Journal of Clinical Oncology, 12*, 2621–2629.

Cancer Statistics. (1997). http://www.cancer.org/eprise/main.docroot/STT/stt_0_1997

Draper, G. J., Sanders, B. M., & Kinston, J. E. (1986). Second primary neoplasms in patients with retinoblastoma. *Br. J. Cancer, 53*, 661–666.

Espy, K. A., Moore, I. M., Kaufmann, P. M., Kramer, J. H., Matthay, K., & Hutter, J. J. (2001). Chemotherapeutic CNS prophylaxis and neuropsychologic change in children with acute lymphoblastic leukemia: A prospective study. *Journal of Pediatric Psychology, 26*(1), 1–9.

Ettinger, D. S. (1995). Preventing chemotherapy-induced nausea and vomiting: An update on a review of emesis. *Seminars in Oncology, 22*, 4:10, 6–18.

Feingold, L., Savitz, D. A., & John, E. M. (1992). Use of a job-exposure matrix to evaluate parental occupation and childhood cancer. *Cancer Causes and Control, 3*, 161–169.

Feychting, M., Schulgen, G., Olsen, J. H., & Ahlbom, A. (1995). Magnetic fields and childhood cancer—a pooled analysis of two Scandinavian studies. *European Journal of Cancer, 31A*(12), 2035–2039.

Ford, C., Whitlock, J. A., & Pietsch, J. B. (1997). Glutamine-supplemented tube feedings versus total parenteral nutrition in children receiving intensive chemotherapy. *Journal of Pediatric Oncology Nursing, 14*(2), 68–72.

Greenlee, R. T., Murray, T., Bolden, S., & Wingo, P. A. (2000). Cancer statistics, 2000. *CA: A Cancer Journal for Clinicians, 50*(1), 7–34.

Gurney, J. G., Davis, S., Severson, R. K., Fang, J. Y., Ross, J. A., & Robison (1996). Trends in cancer incidence among children in the U.S. *Cancer, 78*(3), 532–541.

Haase, J. E., & Rostad, M. (1994). Experiences of completing cancer therapy: Children's perspectives. *Oncology Nursing Forum, 21*(9), 1483–1494.

Haupt, R., Fears, T., Robinson, L., et al. (1994). Educational attainment in long-term survivors of childhood acute lymphoblastic leukemia. *Journal of the American Medical Association, 272*, 1427–1432.

Hinds, P. S. (1988). Adolescent hopefulness in illness and health. *Advances in Nursing Science, 10*(3), 79–88.

Hockenberry-Eaton, M., Dilorio, C., & Kemp, V. (1995). The relationship of illness longevity and relapse with self-perception, cancer stressors, anxiety, and coping strategies in children with cancer. *Journal of Pediatric Oncology Nursing, 12*(2), 71–79.

Hockenberry-Eaton, M., Hinds, P. S., Alcoser, P., O'Neill, J. B., Euell, K., Gattuso, J., & Taylor, J. (1998). Fatigue in children and adolescents with cancer. *Journal of Pediatric Oncology Nursing, 15*(3), 172–182.

Hockenberry-Eaton, M., Kemp, V., & DiIorio, C. (1994). Cancer stressors and protective factors: Predictors of stress experienced during treatment for childhood cancer. *Research in Nursing and Health, 17*, 351–361.

Hollen, P. J., & Hobbie, W. L. (1996). Decision making and risk behaviors of cancer-surviving adolescents and their peers. *Journal of Pediatric Oncology Nursing, 13*(3), 121–134.

Hum, M. C., & Kamen, B. A. (1996). Folate, antifolates, and folate analogs in pediatric oncology. *Investigational New Drugs, 14*, 101–111.

Jankovic, M., Brouwers, P., Valsecchi, M. G., et al. (1994). Association of 1800 cGy cranial irradiation with intellectual function in children with acute lymphoblastic leukaemia. *The Lancet, 344*, 224–227.

Kaufmann, P. M., Moore, I. M., Espy, K. A., & Hutter, J. J. (1996). The late effects of triple intrathecal chemotherapy on neuropsychological outcome at 24 months post leukemia diagnosis. *Journal of the International Neuropsychological Society, (Conference Proceedings) 42*.

Kornblith, A. B., Herndon II, J. E., Zuckerman, E., Cella, D. E., Cherin, E., Wolchok, S., Weiss, R. B., Diehl, L. F., Henderson, E., Cooper, M. R., Schiffer, C., Canellos, G. P., Mayer, R. J., Silver, R. T., Schilling, A., Peterson, B. A., Greenberg, D., & Holland, J. C. (1998). Comparison of psychological adaptation of advanced stage Hodgkin's disease and acute leukemia survivors. *Annals of Oncology, 9*, 297–306.

Kramer, S., Ward, E., Meadows, A. T., et al. (1987). Medical and drug risk factors associated with neuroblastoma: Case-control study. *Journal National Cancer Institute, 78*, 797–804.

Layfield, L. J., Thompson, J. K., Dodge, R. K., & Kerns, B. J. (1995). Prognostic indicators for neuroblastoma: Stage, grade, DNA ploidy, MIB-1-proliferation index, p53, HER-2/neu and EGFr—A survival study. *Journal of Surgical Oncology, 59*, 21–27.

Leiss, J. K., & Savitz, D. A. (1995). Home pesticide use and childhood cancer: A case-control study. *American Journal of Public Health, 85*(2), 249–252.

Lukens, J. N. (1994). Progress resulting from clinical trials. *Cancer Supplement, 74*(9), 2710–2718.

Mackie, E., Hill, J., Kondryn, H., & McNalley, R. (2000). Adult psychosocial outcomes in long-term survivors of acute lymphoblastic leukaemia and Wilms' tumour: A controlled study. *Lancet, 355*, 1310–1314.

Malkin, D., & Portwine, C. (1994). The genetics of childhood cancer. *European Journal of Cancer, 30A*(13), 1942–1946.

Malvy, D. J. M., Arnaud, J., Burtschy, B., Sommelet, D., Leverger, G., Dostalova, L., & Amédée-Manesme, O. (1997). Antioxidant micronutrients and childhood malignancy during oncological treatment. *Medical and Pediatric Oncology, 29,* 213–217.

Malvy, D. J. M., Burtschy, B., Arnaud, J., Sommelet, D., Leverger, G., Dostalova, L., Drucker, J., & Amédée-Manesme, O. (1993). Serum beta-carotene and antioxidant micronutrients in children with cancer. *International Journal of Epidemiology, 22*(5), 761–771.

Martin, P. L., Look, A. T., Schnell, S., Harris, M. B., Pullen, J., Shuster, J. J., Carroll, A. J., Pettenati, M. J., & Rao, P. N. (1996). Comparison of fluorescence in situ hybridization, cytogenetic analysis, and DNA index analysis to detect chromosomes 4 and 10 aneuploidy in pediatric acute lymphoblastic leukemia: A pediatric oncology group study. *Journal of Pediatric Hematology/Oncology, 18*(2), 113–121.

Miller, R. W., Young, J. L., & Novakovic, B. (1995). Childhood cancer. *Cancer Supplement, 75*(1), 395–405.

Mollova, N., Moore, I. M., Hutter, J., & Schram, K. (1995). Fast atom bombardment mass spectrometry of phospholipids in human cerebral spinal fluid. *Biological Mass Spectrometry, 30,* 1405–1420.

Mooney, K. H. (1993). Biologic basis of childhood cancer. In G. V. Foley, D. Fochtman, & K. H. Mooney (Eds.), *Nursing care of the child with cancer* (pp. 25–55). Philadelphia: W. B. Saunders Company.

Moore, I. M. (1995). Central nervous system toxicity of cancer therapy in children: State of the science. *Journal of the Association of Pediatric Oncology Nursing, 12,* 203–210.

Moore, I. M., Espy, K. A., Kaufmann, P., Kramer, J., Kaemingk, K., Miketova, P., Mollova, N., Kaspar, M., Pasgovel, A., Schram, K., Wara, W., Hutter, J., & Matthay, K. (2000). A research program investigating cognitive consequences of treatment for childhood ALL: Cell membrane damage and intellectual and academic abilities in children receiving central nervous system treatment. *Seminars in Oncology Nursing, 16,* 279–290.

Moore, I., Kramer, J., Wara, W., & Ablin, A. (1991). Cognitive function in children with leukemia: Effect of radiation dose and time since irradiation. *Cancer, 68,* 1913–1917.

Mott, M. G. (1995). Neoplasia in childhood—25 years of progress. *Annals of Oncology, 6*(Suppl. 1), 3–9.

Mulhern, R., Fairclough, D., & Ochs, J. (1991). A prospective comparison of neuropsychologic performance of children surviving leukemia who received 18-Gy, 24-Gy or no cranial irradiation. *Journal of Clinical Oncology, 9,* 1348–1356.

Mulhern, R. K., Wasserman, A. L., Friedman, A. G., Faircough, D., & Ochs, J. (1989). Social competence and behavioral adjustment of children who are long-term survivors of cancer. *Pediatrics, 83*(1), 18–25.

Mulhern, R. K., Tyc, V. L., Phipps, S., Crom, D., Barclay, D., Greenwald, C., Hudson, M., & Thompson, I. E. (1995). Health-related behaviors of survivors of childhood cancer. *Medical and Pediatric Oncology, 25,* 159–165.

Mulhern, R., Wasserman, A., Fairclough, D., & Ochs, J. (1988). Memory function in disease-free survivors of childhood acute lymphocytic leukemia given CNS prophylaxis with or without 1,800 cGy cranial radiation. *Journal of Clinical Oncology, 6*(2), 315–320.

Ochs, J., Mulhern, R., Fairclough, D., Parvey, L., Whitaker, J., Chlien, L. N., Mauer, A., & Simone, J. (1991). Comparison of neuropsychologic functioning and clinical indicators of neurotoxicity in long-term survivors of childhood leukemia given cranial radiation or parenteral methotrexate: A prospective study. *Journal of Clinical Oncology, 9,* 145–151.

Prassopoulos, P., Cavouras, D., Golfinopoulos, S., Evlogias, N., Theodoropoulos, V., & Panagiotou, J. (1996). Quantitative assessment of cerebral atrophy during and after treatment in children with acute lymphoblastic leukemia. *Investigative Radiology, 31*(12), 749–754.

Ries, L. A. G., Smith, M. A., Gurney, J. G., Linet, M., Tamara, T., & Young, J. L. (Eds.). (1999). Cancer incidence and survival among children and adolescents: United States SEER program 1975–1995. National Cancer Institute SEER Program. NIH Pub. No. 99–4649. Bethesda, MD: U.S. Department of Health and Human Services.

Rivera, G. K., Raimondi, S. C., Hancock, M. L., et al. (1991). Improved outcome in childhood acute lymphoblastic leukaemia with reinforced early treatment and rotational combination chemotherapy. *Lancet, 337,* 61–66.

Robison, L. L., Buckley, J. D., & Bunin, G. (1995). Assessment of environmental and genetic factors in the etiology of childhood cancers: The children's cancer group epidemiology program. *Environmental Health Perspectives, 103*(6), 111–116.

Rubinitz, J. E., & Crist, W. M. (1997). Molecular genetics of childhood cancer: Implications for pathogenesis, diagnosis, and treatment. *Pediatrics, 100*(1), 101–108.

Sawyer, M. G., Toogood, I., Rice, M., Haskell, C., & Baghurst, P. (1988). School performance and psychological adjustment of children treated for leukemia—A long-term follow-up. *The American Journal of Pediatric Hematology/Oncology, 11*(2), 146–152.

Schwartz, C. L., Hobbie, W. L., Constine, L. S., & Ruccione, K. S. (1994). *Survivors of childhood cancer.* Mosby-Year Book, Inc.

Schwartzbaum, J. A. (1992). Influence of the mother's prenatal drug consumption on risk of neuroblastoma in the child. *American Journal of Epidemiology, 135*(12), 1358–1367.

Seibel, N. L., & Reaman, G. H. (1996). New microtubular agents in pediatric oncology. *Investigational New Drugs, 14,* 49–54.

Shu, X. O., Reaman, G. H., Lampin, B., Sather, H. N., Pendergrass, T. W., & Robison, L. L. (1994). Association of paternal diagnostic X-ray exposure with risk of infant leukemia. *Cancer Epidemiology, Biomarkers and Prevention, 30,* 645–653.

Shu, X. O., Ross, J. A., Pendergrass, T. W., Reaman, G. H., Lampkin, B., & Robison, L. L. (1996). Parental alcohol consumption, cigarette smoking, and risk of infant leukemia: A children's cancer group study. *Journal of the National Cancer Institute, 88*(1), 24–31.

Sloper, T., Larcombe, I. J., & Charlton, A. (1994). Psychosocial adjustment of five-year survivors of childhood cancer. *Journal of Cancer Education, 9*(3), 163–169.

Suita, S., Zaisen, Y., Sera, Y., Takamatsu, H., Mizote, H., Ohgami, H., Kurosaki, N., Ueda, K., Tasaka, H., Miyazaki, S., Sugimoto, T., Kawakami, K., Tsuneyoshi, M., Yano, H., Akiyama, H., & Ikeda, K. (1996). Mass screening for neuroblastoma: Quo vadis? A 9-year experience from the pediatric oncology study group of the Kyushu area in Japan. *Journal of Pediatric Surgery, 3*(4), 555–558.

Trueworthy, R., Shuster, J., Look, T., Crist, W., Borowitz, M., Carroll, A., Frankel, L., Harris, M., Wagner, H., Haggard, M., et al. (1992). Ploidy of lymphoblasts is the strongest predictor of treatment outcome in B-progenitor cell acute lymphoblastic leukemia in childhood: A pediatric oncology group study. *Journal of Clinical Oncology, 10*, 606–613.

Tyc, V. L., Mulhern, R. K., Jayawardene, D., & Fairclough, D. (1995a). Chemotherapy-induced nausea and emesis in pediatric cancer patients: An analysis of coping strategies. *Journal of Pain and Symptom Management, 10*(5), 338–347.

Tyc, V. L., Vallelunga, L., Mahoney, S., Smith, B. F., & Mulhern, R.K. (1995b). Nutritional and treatment-related characteristics of pediatric oncology patients referred or not referred for nutritional support. *Medical and Pediatric Oncology, 25*, 379–388.

Varni, J. W., Katz, E. R., Colegrove, D., & Dolgin, M. (1994a). Perceived social support and adjustment of children with newly diagnosed cancer. *Developmental and Behavioral Pediatrics, 15*(1), 20–26.

Varni, J. W., Katz, E. R., Colegrove, R., & Dolgin, M. (1994b). Perceived stress and adjustment of long-term survivors of childhood cancer. *Journal of Psychosocial Oncology, 12*(3), 1–17.

van Eys, J. (1991). The truly cured child? *Pediatrician, 18*, 90–95.

Yeazel, M. W., Buckley, J. D., Woods, W. G., Ruccione, K., & Robison, L. L. (1995). History of maternal fetal loss and increased risk of childhood acute leukemia at an early age. *Cancer, 75*(7), 1718–1727.

Zahm, S. H., & Devesa, S. S. (1995). *Environmental Health Perspectives, 103*(6), 177–184.

CHAPTER 5

Cardiovascular Responsivity to Stress and Preclinical Manifestations of Cardiovascular Disease in Youth

Frank A. Treiber, Harry Davis, and J. Rick Turner

D espite declines over the past several decades, cardiovascular disease (CVD) continues to be the leading cause of death in adults in the United States (American Heart Association, 2000). Essential Hypertension (EH), a major risk factor for CVD, remains high in the U.S., affecting approximately 50 million adults (Burt, Whelton, Roccella, Brown, Cutler, Higgins, Horan, & Labarthe, 1995; Hypertension Detection and Follow-up Program Cooperative Group, 1984). Invasive (e.g., angioplasty, coronary artery bypass) and pharmacologic interventions often prove extremely expensive, and adherence problems are an issue with lifestyle and pharmacologic regimens (National High Blood Pressure Education Program, 1993; Whelton, He, & Appel, 1996). Therefore, treatment of CVD often proves very expensive and difficult for the patients to adhere to. Effective primary prevention of CVD would decrease the risk of premature CVD, thus eliminating hundreds of millions of dollars of health care costs and increasing individuals longevity and quality of life (Alpert, Murphy, & Treiber, 1994; Whelton, He, & Appel, 1996).

Necropsy studies have established that the pathogenesis of CVD can be traced to childhood (Berenson, Wattigney, Tracy, Newman, Srinivasan, Webber, Dalferes, & Strong, 1992; Newman, Freedman, Voors, Gard, Srinivasan, Cresanta, Williamson, Webber, & Berenson, 1986; PDAY Research Group, 1990). Thus, preventive efforts might prove more successful if begun during childhood rather than in early to middle adulthood, by which time many pathobiologic alterations related to CVD have already occurred (Alpert, Murphy, & Treiber, 1994; Strong, Deckelbaum, Gidding, Kavey, Washington, Wilmore, & Perry, 1992; Strong & Kelder, 1996). Early pediatric epidemiologic studies focused upon the development of traditional physical CVD risk factors (e.g., blood pressure (BP), adiposity, cholesterol subfractions) and their relationships to behavioral lifestyle factors that have been associated with CVD in adults (e.g., diet, physical activity, smoking, and Type A behavior pattern (Arbeit, Johnson, & Mot, 1992; Berenson, 1986; Berenson, McMahan, Voors, Webber, Srinivasan, Frank, Foster, & Blonde, 1980; Strong & Kelder, 1996). Based in part upon these findings, a number of weight reduction and/or physical activity enhancement studies have been conducted using case study, small group, family, and recently, school-based approaches. These studies have met with mixed results in altering physical CVD risk factors (e.g., cholesterol, BP, and percent body fat) (Alpert, Murphy, & Treiber, 1994; Resnicow, 1993). These findings suggest not only the need for further refinement of such interventions, but also the possibility that other behavioral factors may need to be targeted.

DEFINITION AND RATIONALE OF CARDIOVASCULAR RESPONSIVITY (CVR)

A behavioral factor that has been posited as a candidate risk factor for CVD is exaggerated cardiovascular responsivity (CVR) to stress (Fredrikson & Matthews, 1990; Manuck, 1994; Manuck, Kasprowicz, & Muldoon, 1990). CVR can be defined as the magnitude and pattern of an individual's physiological responsivity resulting from exposure to a discrete environmental stimulus (Matthews, Weiss, Detre, Dembroski, Falkner, Manuck, & Williams, 1986; Sherwood & Turner, 1995). Findings (predominantly involving adults) have long shown that such responses may vary considerably among individuals. It has been proposed that perhaps exaggerated CV responsivity to such challenges may play a role in the development or expression of CVD including coronary heart disease (CHD) and EH (Krantz & Manuck, 1984). There have been a number of review articles, monographs, and books written about CVR in animals, adults, and youth (Manuck, 1994; Matthews, Weiss, Detre, Dembroski, Falkner, Manuck, & Williams, 1986; Murphy, 1992; Sallis, Dimsdale, & Caine, 1988; Schneiderman, Weiss, & Kaufman, 1989; Turner, 1994). Thus, this chapter is not meant to be a review of the entire field. Rather, the purpose is to provide an overview of CVR in youth, with particular emphasis on its relationships to preclinical markers of CVD risk. We then propose a biobehavioral reactivity model that depicts several pathways by which exaggerated CVR may eventually lead to overt manifestations of CVD.

The rationale for evaluating CVR is twofold. First, unique information (e.g., BP response to a stressor) can be obtained that is not accessible via a standard evaluation (e.g., resting BP during a clinical examination). Second, this information can be helpful in understanding the pathophysiology of CVD, and in the development of effective prevention and treatment programs. Recent findings indicated that BP responses to mental stress were stronger predictors of future silent ischemia than BP at rest and in response to treadmill exercise in post myocardial infarction patients (Jiang, Babyak, Krantz, Waugh, Coleman, Hanson, Fied, McNulty, Morris, O'Connor, & Blumenthal, 1996). Whether CVR studies will warrant becoming a standard part of diagnostic screenings for identification of CVD risk and/or treatment, however, requires further scientific evaluation.

Stability of CVR

A crucial assumption of CVR researchers is that CVR responsivity is a stable individual difference characteristic, consistent across time (i.e., temporal stability) and stressors (i.e., intertask consistency) (Manuck, Kasprowicz, & Muldoon, 1990; Matthews, Weiss, Detre, Dembroski, Falkner, Manuck, & Williams, 1986; Turner, 1994). If CVR to stress plays a role in the prediction of CVD, such consistency is a prerequisite and should be established relatively early in life (Murphy, 1992).

Temporal Stability of CVR

Twenty-eight years is the longest time interval studied to date (in adults or youth), in which cold pressor reactivity was assessed on 151 subjects from a cohort initially 6–19 years old (Barnett, Hines Jr., Schirger, & Gage, 1963). All 31 subjects in the follow-up sample who had originally been classified as hyperreactive (systolic BP [SBP] increase > 20 mmHg) were still classified as hyperreactive at follow up, and 99 of the 120 normoreactive subjects retained their initial classification.

Since that time a number of pediatric researchers have evaluated stability of BP, heart rate (HR), and most recently, cardiac output (CO) and total peripheral resistance (TPR) (the underlying hemodynamic regulators of BP control) across periods of time ranging from 1 week to 6 years (Giordani, Manuck, & Farmer, 1981; Mahoney, Schieken, Clarke, & Lauer, 1988; Matthews, Rakaczky, Stoney, & Manuck, 1987; Matthews, Woodall, & Stoney, 1990; McGrath & O'Brien, 2001; Murphy, Alpert, & Walker, 1992; Murphy, Alpert, Walker, & Willey, 1994; Murphy, Alpert, Willey, & Somes, 1988; Murphy, Stoney, Alpert, & Walker, 1995; Taras & Sallis, 1992; Treiber, Raunikar, Davis, Fernandez, Levy, & Strong, 1994). In general, these researchers have shown that, regardless of gender and ethnicity, CVR is stable in youth for a variety of stressors, including video game challenge, postural change, cold pressor, isometric handgrip, mirror image tracing, and mental arithmetic. Stability coefficients are comparable to those observed for resting BP and HR, particularly when absolute stressor response levels are used (r range = 0.40–0.70) (Mahoney, Schieken, Clarke, & Lauer, 1988; Matthews, Rakaczky, Stoney, & Manuck, 1987). When change scores are used, there tends to be a decrease in the correlation coefficients that is comparable to findings in adults (Sherwood & Turner, 1995; Turner, 1994). The lower stability coefficients for change scores are expected since the change score contains potential measurement error of both the baseline measure and of the response measure. Recently, Kamarck, Jennings, Debski, Glickman-Weiss, Johnson, Eddy, and Manuck (1992); Kamarck, Jennings, Stewart, and Eddy (1993); Manuck, Kamarck, Kasprowicz, and Waldstein (1993) have shown that aggregating adults' CV responses to comparable behavioral stressors increases the temporal stability coefficients of change scores (r range = 0.85–0.96). Such approaches may also prove useful in CVR studies involving youth.

Intertask Consistency of CVR

The other underlying assumption of CVR research is that an individual who is hyperreactive to one stressor (e.g., cold pressor) is likely to exhibit similar hemodynamic response changes to other stressors (e.g., speech preparation). Similarly to adult studies, of the few studies conducted with youth, the majority of researchers have assessed BP and HR responses and observed moderate consistency across a variety of stressor comparisons (Strong, Miller,

Striplin, & Salehbhai, 1978; Taras & Sallis, 1992; Verhaaren, Schieken, Mosteller, Hewitt, Eaves, & Nance, 1991). For instance, Parker, Croft, Cresanta, Freedman, Burke, Webber, and Berenson (1987) observed intertask correlations of peak BP responses from 0.53–0.84 to hand cold pressor, isometric handgrip exercise, and postural change. Matthews, Rakaczky, Stoney, and Manuck (1987) observed consistency in BP and HR change scores to mental arithmetic, mirror image tracing, and isometric handgrip exercise (r range = 0.30–0.60). Musante, Raunikar, Treiber, Davis, Dysart, Levy, and Strong (1994) examined the consistency of children's BP, CO, and TPR change scores to postural change, forehead cold, and a challenging video game (Atari Breakout). The highest coefficients across stressors were noted for CO and TPR (r range = 0.32–0.68). These findings, along with those of McGrath and O'Brien (2001), suggest that intertask consistency is comparable or may be higher for the underlying hemodynamic regulators of BP control (i.e., CO and TPR) compared to BP responses, particularly diastolic responses, and are consistent with recent adult findings (Sherwood & Turner, 1995; Turner, Sherwood, & Light, 1994).

CVR in the Laboratory Versus the Field

Another assumption of laboratory-based CVR research is that individuals who are hyperresponsive in the lab will also be hyperresponsive to naturally occurring stressors in the free-living environment. The advent of ambulatory BP monitoring has permitted such evaluations to be conducted. However, of the few studies conducted in youth, low to moderate relationships have been observed between CVR to laboratory stressors and ambulatory BP measurements in various field settings (Coates, Parker, & Kolodner, 1982; Ewart & Kolodner, 1993; Langewitz, Ruddel, Schachinger, & Schmieder, 1989). For example, Matthews, Manuck, and Saab (1986) found that teenagers classified as being hyperreactive to serial subtraction, isometric handgrip exercise, and star tracing also exhibited elevated CV responses while giving a speech at school. Twenty-four-hour ambulatory BP in youth was found to correlate significantly with BP responses to a variety of stressors (i.e., postural change, video game, forehead cold, and dynamic exercise) (Treiber, Murphy, Davis, Raunikar, Pflieger, & Strong, 1994). Researchers who completed a longitudinal study found that in addition to the contributions of anthropometrics, demographics, and resting BP, BP and/or TPR responses to a behavioral challenge (i.e., video game) and to postural change (supine to standing position) were predictive of 24-hr ambulatory BP 2 years later in children with family histories of EH (Del Rosario, Treiber, Harshfield, Davis, & Strong, 1998). Collectively, these recent findings are promising with regard to the potential value of laboratory based CVR studies in predicting CV functioning in the free-living environment, particularly given the lack of control over various moderating influences upon BP (e.g., posture, physical activity, affective state, etc.) (Manuck, Kasprowicz, & Muldoon, 1990).

BIOBEHAVIORAL CVR STRESS MODEL

In summary, CVR to behavioral challenges in the laboratory is a stable individual difference dimension in childhood, as noted by its relative stability over time and across challenges. Further, there is an indication that CVR in the lab may be representative of CVR in the natural setting. Given these conclusions, and the findings in adults suggesting associations between CVR and various manifestations of CVD (including EH and CHD) using case control, retrospective designs, and a few prospective studies (Fredrikson & Matthews, 1990; Manuck, 1994; Manuck, Kasprowicz, & Muldoon, 1990; Schneiderman, 1987), a biobehavioral stress responsivity model is proposed. Two primary pathways are identified (i.e., vascular and ventricular remodeling) whereby CVR may contribute to the initiation and pathogenic progression of CVD. The model identifies expected relationships between CVR and changes in preclinical markers of CVD (e.g., increased BP, increased left ventricular mass (LVM), concentric remodeling, and decreased endothelial dependent arterial dilation) prior to overt manifestation of EH or CHD. A diagram of the biobehavioral CVR stress model and hypothesized pathogenic changes in preclinical markers of CVD is presented in Figure 5.1. This model is not meant to be comprehensive, as other possible mechanistic pathways may also link CVR with CVD (e.g., renin-angiotensin system, sodium sensitivity, catecholamine responsivity (Schneiderman & Skyler, 1996; Turner, 1994).

Individual differences in the magnitude of CVR are influenced by a multitude of variables, which can be categorized into one of two primary grouping factors. The first group reflects an underlying response potential, the second consists of constitutional factors (Manuck, Morrison, Bellack, & Polefrone, 1985). Important markers of response potential include genetics (e.g., positive family history of CVD), ethnicity, and gender. Examples of constitutional factors that have been associated with resting BP and/or CVR in children, adolescents, and/or young adults include pubertal level, adiposity, chronic environmental stress, aerobic fitness, and coping styles (e.g., anger suppres-

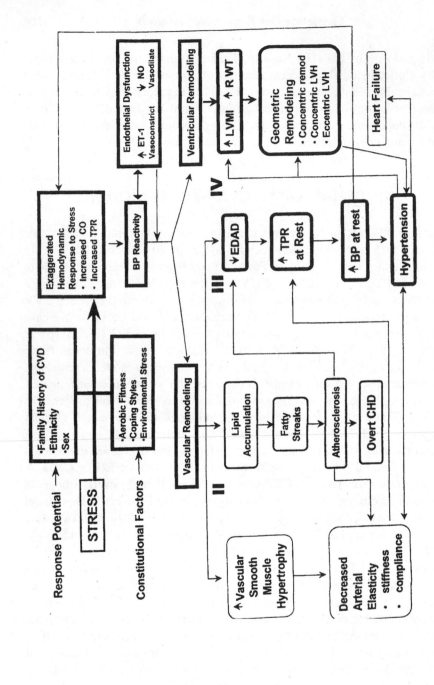

FIGURE 5.1 Diagram of cardiovascular responsivity to stress and its potential impact on cardiovascular health.

sion/expression, John Henryism, family functioning (Anderson, McNeilly, & Myers, 1991; Gutin, Manos, Manghram, Thompson, & Treiber, 1993; James, Harinett, & Kalsbeek, 1983; Johnson, Schork, & Spielberger, 1987; Johnson, Spielberger, Worden, & Jacobs, 1987; Light, 1989; Manuck, Morrison, Bellack, & Polefrone, 1985; Murphy, Alpert, Willey, Christman, Sexton, & Harshfield, 1989; Murphy, Alpert, Willey, & Somes, 1988; Murphy, Stoney, Alpert, & Walker, 1995; Musante, Turner, Treiber, Davis, & Strong, 1996; Pflieger, Treiber, Davis, McCaffrey, Raunikar, & Strong, 1994; Wright, Treiber, Davis, Strong, Levy, Van Huss, & Batchelor, 1993; Wright, Treiber, Davis, & Strong, 1997).

As depicted in Figure 5.1, an individual's CV stress responses are influenced by inherent response potential (e.g., family history of CVD, ethnicity, gender) and moderated by constitutional factors. Complex neuroendocrine changes occur, characterized by increased sympathetic arousal, activating the CV system, and increasing CO and/or TPR, with subsequent elevation of BP (Folkow, 1990a, 1990b; Folkow, Grimby, & Thulesius, 1958; Schneiderman, 1987; Sherwood & Turner, 1995). These altered hemodynamic forces result in increases in cardiac and vascular wall tension and intravascular shear stress (Folkow, 1990; Folkow, Grimby, & Thulesius, 1958). Recurrent and/or sustained exaggerated stress-induced increases of vascular and ventricular wall tension may lead to secondary CV structural adaptation (i.e., vascular remodeling and ventricular remodeling) to help normalize wall tension (Folkow, 1990; Folkow, 1990; Folkow, Grimby, & Thulesius, 1958).

Recurrent stress-induced alterations of hemodynamic forces may also result in endothelial dysfunction, a relatively early event in the pathogenesis of CV disease (Davies, Barbee, Lal, Robotewskyj, & Griem, 1995; Luscher & Vanhoutte, 1990; Panza, Casino, Kilcoyne, & Quyyumi, 1993). Endothelial damage causes an enhanced endothelial permeability to plasma lipoproteins, an increased platelet adherence, and functional imbalances in local pro- and antithrombotic factors, and in the release of growth stimulators, inhibitors, and vasoactive substances (Davies, Barbee, Lal, Robotewskyj, & Griem, 1995; Gimbrone, Cybulsky, Kume, Collins, & Resnick, 1995; Luscher & Vanhoutte, 1990). The functional imbalances in vasoactive substances resulting from endothelial damage include decreased effectiveness of endothelial-derived relaxing factors (e.g., nitric oxide) due to decreased production, and more rapid inactivation of such factors and/or decreased sensitivity of smooth muscle to such factors (Luscher & Vanhoutte, 1990; Panza, Casino, Kilcoyne, & Quyyumi, 1993; Taddei, Virdis, Mattei, Ghiadoni, Sudano, & Salvetti, 1996). Related to this imbalance, an increase occurs in endothelial release of the potent vasoconstrictive peptide endothelin-1 (ET-1) in response to physiologic stimuli related to humoral (e.g., thrombin, angiotensin II) and physical (e.g., transmural pressure, flow, and shear stress) factors (Davies, Barbee, Lal, Robotewskyj, & Griem, 1995; Lemne, Lundeberg, Theodorsson, & de Faire, 1994). To date, simple well validated noninvasive markers of nitric oxide function have not been developed. Accordingly, invasive intraarterial pharmacologic challenges (e.g., nitrous prusside, acetylcholine) are required to assess nitric oxide function.

Endothelial dysfunction, particularly the vasoconstrictive actions of ET-1, is thought to play a role in the development of ventricular remodeling and vascular remodeling (Andrawis, Wang, & Abernethy, 1996; Gimbrone, Cybulsky, Kume, Collins, & Resnick, 1995; Ichikawa, Hidai, Okuda, Kimata, Matsuoka, Hosoda, Quertermous, & Kawana, 1996; Luscher & Vanhoutte, 1990; Weber, Sun, & Guarda, 1994). Ventricular remodeling includes increased LVM and/or relative wall thickness (RWT) and adverse LV geometry (concentric remodeling, eccentric or concentric LV hypertrophy), all of which are independent predictors of CV morbidity, mortality, and heart failure (Casale, Devereux, Milner, Zullo, Harshfield, Pickering, & Laragh, 1986; Koren, Devereux, Casale, Savage, & Laragh, 1991).

An early functional manifestation of vascular remodeling is diminished endothelium dependent arterial vasodilation (EDAD) to reactive hyperemia (Celermajer, Sorensen, Barley, Jeffrey, Carter, & Deanfield, 1994; Celermajer, Sorensen, Bull, Robinson, & Deanfield, 1994; Celermajer, Sorensen, Georgakopoulos, Bull, Thomas, Robinson, & Deanfield, 1993; Celermajer, Sorensen, Gooch, Spiegelhalter, Miller, Sullivan, Lloyd, & Vernfield, 1992), depicted in Arm III of Figure 5.1. Manifestations of vascular remodeling also include vascular smooth muscle hypertrophy and increases in collagen deposition, which eventually leads to decreased arterial elasticity. The vascular remodeling process also involves development of fatty streaks and advanced lesions. These structural alterations eventually decrease arterial elasticity, exacerbate plaque formation, and enhance the atherosclerotic process leading to coronary heart disease (Folkow, 1990a, 1990b; Folkow, Grimby, & Thulesius, 1958; Schneiderman, 1987). These latter changes are depicted in Arms I & II of Figure 5.1.

Collectively, these morphological and functional alterations are hypothesized to lead to elevations in resting TPR and BP. This leads to further increases in LVM, relative wall thickness, and BP reactivity. A vicious cycle ensues that contributes to the pathogenesis of EH and CHD. Although this model has received some empirical support (briefly reviewed below), definitive evidence to support the etiologic role of reactivity in the development of CHD is still lacking and needs to be tested in a prospective manner. Following is a synopsis of CVR findings in youth which support the proposed model.

RESPONSE POTENTIAL AND CVR

Family History of CVD and CVR

Epidemiologic researchers have consistently found certain groups of individuals to be at increased risk for development of CVD (e.g., males, African Americans, individuals with family history of CVD) (Burt, Whelton, Roccella, Brown, Cutler, Higgins, Horan, & Labarthe, 1995; Genest, Koiw, & Kuchel, 1977; Gillum, 1991). Interestingly, although not entirely consistent, these groups are prone to exhibit exaggerated CVR.

A positive family history of essential hypertension has been associated with an increased risk of development of EH (Genest, Koiw, & Kuchel, 1977; Platt, 1967; Stamler, Stamler, Riedlinger, Algera, & Roberts, 1979). Likewise, family history of premature myocardial infarction (i.e., < 55 years of age in biologic parents and/or grandparents) has been associated with increased risk of development of CHD (Nora, Lortscher, Spangler, Nora, & Kimberling, 1980; Roncaglioni, Santoro, D'Avanzo, Negri, Nobili, Ahedda, Pietropaolo, Franzosi, LaVecchia, & Feruglio, 1992). If CVR is associated with CVD, it might be anticipated that a positive family history of CHD or EH would be associated with greater CVR. Research in youth (Musante, Treiber, Strong, & Levy, 1990; Treiber, McCaffrey, Pflieger, Raunikar, Strong, & Davis, 1993; Treiber, Strong, Arensman, Forrest, Davis, & Musante, 1991) and young adults (Falkner, Kushner, Onesti, & Angelakos, 1981; Fredrikson & Matthews, 1990; Manuck, Kasprowicz, & Muldoon, 1990) has indicated that a family history of EH or premature CVD is often associated with increased CVR to stress. The original work of Hines (1937a) indicated that 95.4% of children were hyperreactors if both parents had EH, while 43.4% were hyperreactors if only one parent had EH. A meta-analysis performed by Matthews et al. (1993) indicated that a family history of EH is associated with greater BP responsivity to stress. The majority of the studies evaluated involved young adults.

Several studies published since that time involving children and adolescents have corroborated and extended the conclusions of that meta-analysis. For example, boys with a family history of EH (defined as one or both biologic parents and one or more biologic grandparents with physician verified EH) exhibited greater TPR at rest and in response to the laboratory stressors of video game challenge and forehead cold stimulation than with negative family history cohorts (Treiber, McCaffrey, Musante, Rhodes, Davis, Strong, & Levy, 1993). African American males with a family history of premature myocardial infarction (MI) or EH have exhibited greater SBP increases to supine cycle ergometry or cold stimulation due to greater TPR responsivity than negative family history peers (Musante, Treiber, Strong, & Levy, 1990; Treiber, McCaffrey, Strong, Davis, & Baranowski, 1991). Collectively, these findings indicate that a family history of CVD is often associated with exaggerated CVR in children and adults.

Ethnicity and CVR

African Americans have a greater prevalence of EH than whites (Akinkubge, 1985; Burt, Whelton, Roccella, Brown, Cutler, Higgins, Horan, & Labarthe, 1995). Classification of ethnicity is used to designate sociocultural frameworks within which any ethnic CVR differences are thought to be due to combinations of differences in sociocultural experiences and biologic/genetic factors (Anderson, McNeilly, & Myers, 1991; Light, Turner, Hinderliter, & Sherwood, 1993). A number of investigators have examined the potential role of exaggerated CVR to stress as an underlying mechanism related to these ethnic differences in EH (Anderson, McNeilly, & Myers, 1991; Light, Turner, Hinderliter, & Sherwood, 1993; Saab, Llabre, Hurwitz, Frame, Reineke, Fins, McCalla, Cieply, & Schneiderman, 1992). With regard to youth, although not all studies have observed ethnic differences (Falkner & Kushner, 1989; Matthews, Gump, Block, & Allen, 1997) the work of Alpert, Murphy, and colleagues with 6–16 year-olds has consistently shown that African Americans tend to exhibit greater SBP and/or DBP responses to dynamic exercise and a video game challenge (Alpert, Dover, Booker, Martin, & Strong, 1981; Murphy, 1992; Murphy, Alpert, Moes, & Somes, 1986; Murphy, Alpert, & Walker, 1992; Murphy, Alpert, Walker, & Willey, 1991; Murphy, Alpert, Walker, & Willey, 1994; Murphy, Alpert, Willey, & Somes, 1988). Recent studies using echocardiography or impedance cardiography have indicated that African American youths' propensity for a greater BP responsivity to stress appears to be due to greater increases in, or less attenuation of, TPR to video game challenges, dynamic exercise, the social stressor interview, and forehead cold stimulation (Arensman, Treiber, Gruber, & Strong, 1989;

Dysart, Treiber, Pflieger, Davis, & Strong, 1994; Treiber, McCaffrey, Musante, Rhodes, Davis, Strong, & Levy, 1993; Treiber, McCaffrey, Strong, Davis, & Baranowski, 1991; Treiber, Musante, Braden, Arensman, Strong, Levy, & Leverett, 1990; Treiber, Raunikar, Davis, Fernandez, Levy, & Strong, 1994).

Ambulatory BP studies have indicated that among children and adolescents, African Americans tend to exhibit comparable BP to whites while awake but show less decline in BP during sleep (Harshfield, Alpert, Willey, Somes, Murphy, & Dupaul, 1989). Recent findings by Treiber and colleagues indicated that among youth with positive family history of EH, African Americans and males exhibited higher BP throughout a 24-hr period than whites and females, respectively (Thompson, Treiber, Johnson, & Davis, 1997; Treiber, Murphy, Davis, Raunikar, Pflieger, & Strong, 1994). Collectively, along with adult findings (Anderson, McNeilly, & Myers, 1991; Light, Turner, Hinderliter, & Sherwood, 1993; Saab, Llabre, Hurwitz, Frame, Reineke, Fins, McCalla, Cieply, & Schneiderman, 1992), it appears that African Americans are more prone to exhibit exaggerated BP responses to laboratory stressors that are predominantly vasoconstrictively mediated.

Gender and CVR

Research with adults has generally found that men exhibit greater SBP responsivity to a wide variety of tasks, including psychomotor, physical performance and speech tasks, than do women (Light, Turner, Hinderliter, & Sherwood, 1993; Matthews, Davis, Stoney, Owens, & Caggiula, 1991; Stoney, Davis, & Matthews, 1987). Relatively few studies involving youth have examined gender differences in reactivity (Matthews, Davis, Stoney, Owens, & Caggiula, 1991; Matthews & Stoney, 1988; Matthews, Woodall, & Stoney, 1990; Murphy, 1992; Murphy, Stoney, Alpert, & Walker, 1995). Collectively, these findings indicate that gender differences, with males exhibiting greater BP reactivity, do not consistently occur until late adolescence to early adulthood. Allen and Matthews (1997) recently conducted an elegant study using impedance cardiography to examine gender differences in prepubertal children and adolescent CVR responsivity to a battery of stressors. Although there were no gender differences in BP responsivity, by adolescence, males exhibited greater vasoconstrictive increases and females exhibited greater CO increases to all four stressors (i.e., forehead cold, mirror tracing, reaction time, and a social competency interview). These findings corroborate recent studies in adults indicating that men's greater BP responsivity appears mediated by greater vasoconstrictive responsivity (i.e., increased TPR) (Girdler, Turner, Sherwood, & Light, 1990; Light, Turner, Hinderliter, & Sherwood, 1993; Sherwood & Turner, 1995).

CONSTITUTIONAL VARIABLES AND CVR

Aerobic Fitness and CVR

Studies with adults have indicated that aerobic fitness may be a buffer against exaggerated CVR (Fillingim & Blumenthal, 1992). This area of research has received relatively little attention in pediatric studies. In two studies, aerobic fitness was associated with decreased BP and HR reactivity to a video game challenge, particularly among African American youths (Alpert, Murphy, & Christman, 1986; Murphy, Alpert, Willey, Christman, Sexton, & Harshfield, 1989). An ambulatory BP monitoring study indicated that aerobically fit youth had lower BP both during the day and at night compared to a cohort of less fit children (Harshfield, Dupaul, Alpert, Christman, Willey, Murphy, & Somes, 1990). Finally, an 8-month exercise training program among hypertensive adolescents resulted in a reduced SBP response to postural change (seated to standing) and submaximal exercise (Hagberg, Goldring, Health, Ehsani, Hernandez, & Holloszy, 1984).

Behavioral Coping Styles and CVR

Several personality and behavioral characteristics, collectively termed behavioral coping styles, have been associated with CVR. The coping style most studied in youth has been the Type A behavior pattern. As in adult studies, findings have been mixed; some studies have revealed positive associations, particularly for SBP responsivity, others have revealed no association, and still others have shown that relationships were moderated by factors such as family history of EH (Alpert & Wilson, 1992). Among a group of adolescents, self-reported anxiety was associated with increased SBP and HR responsivity and chronic outward anger expression was related to increased BP in response to giving a formal speech at school (Matthews, Manuck, & Saab, 1986). Potential for hostility has also been associated with increased BP responsivity to handgrip isometric exercise in teenagers (McCann & Matthews, 1988).

Several indices of family functioning in response to daily stress have received increasing attention in pediatric CVR research. Offspring of parents who characterized their families as being supportive and nurturing exhibited less HR responsivity to isometric handgrip exercise and serial subtraction (Woodall & Matthews, 1989) and lower TPR at rest and in response to forehead cold (Musante, Turner, Treiber, Davis, & Strong, 1996). To our knowledge, only one prospective study has been conducted in this area. Wright, Treiber, Davis, Strong, Levy, Van Huss, and Batchelor (1993) found that maternal ratings of family cohesion (i.e., warmth, and emotional support) and expressiveness (i.e., open expression of feelings and concerns) were associated with lower CVR to postural change and forehead cold stimulation 2 years later in a group of children initially 6–8 years old.

John Henryism (EH) is a coping style characterized by a strong predisposition to confront psychosocial stress in an active and effortful manner. John Henryism has been prospectively associated with the development of EH in African Americans (James, Harinett, & Kalsbeek, 1983). Recently, this coping style was positively related to resting SBP and TPR as well as SBP and TPR responses to forehead cold and postural change and SBP and DBP responses to treadmill exercise in youth who had a family history of EH (Wright, Treiber, Davis, & Strong, 1996).

Chronic Environmental Stress and CVR

Until recently, the role of chronic environmental stress, although hypothesized as contributing to CVD, has rarely been evaluated in youth CVR research. Socioeconomic status (SES) is considered a general proxy for chronic environmental stress. Wright, Treiber, Davis, and Strong (1997) observed that African American and white youths from lower SES environments (i.e., maternal years of education < 12 years) compared to peers from higher SES backgrounds (i.e., maternal years of education > 12 years) exhibited higher BP at rest and during a variety of stressors. This was due to greater vasoconstrictive activity (greater TPR). Using a median split classification of Hollingshead scores, youth from lower SES backgrounds had greater DBP and TPR increases to a reaction time task (Matthews, Gump, Block, & Allen, 1997).

Finally, based upon self-reported severity, consequences, and frequency of interpersonal conflict, youth classified as experiencing high environmental stress exhibited greater DBP and TPR responsivity to a battery of acute lab stressors than to low environmentally stressed peers (Matthews et al., 1997). Interestingly, the influence of SES upon CV function in youth have been found to be moderated by the coping style of John Henryism (Wright et al., 1996). In a sample of youth from low SES environments, those who reported high levels of John Henryism exhibited particularly high TPR at rest and during stress when compared to those low in John Henryism. Further, for youth from the higher SES group, John Henryism scores were unrelated to TPR at rest and during stress. In conclusion, the markers of response potential (i.e., ethnicity, gender, family history of CVD) and the constitutional variables of aerobic fitness, behavioral coping styles, and chronic environmental stress have been shown to have a rather consistent impact upon the CV system of youth through increased TPR mediated BP responsivity to stress.

Preclinical Markers of CVD and CVR

The pathogenesis of CVD follows a relatively consistent progression (Fuster, Badimon, Badimon, & Chesebro, 1992; Ross, 1993; Stary, 1989). Devereux and colleagues have coined the term *preclinical markers* to describe pathogenic changes in cardiovascular structure or function that, if continued, will often progress to overt manifestations of CVD including MI, stroke and EH (Devereux, de Simone, Koren, Roman, & Laragh, 1991; Devereux & Alderman, 1993; Devereux, Koren, de Simone, Roman, & Laragh, 1992). Over the past 10 years an increasing number of research findings have indicated that CVR to acute stressors in the laboratory is associated with various preclinical markers of increased CVD risk both cross sectionally and prospectively.

Prediction of Future CV Functioning

Increased resting BP is a major independent risk factor for CVD, particularly EH (Burt et al., 1995; Hypertension Detection and Follow-up Program Cooperative Group, 1984). Only one study has examined the relationships between CVR in healthy, normotensive youth, and the clinical endpoint of EH in adulthood. Wood, Sheps, Elveback, and Schirger (1984) conducted a 45-year follow-up using the cold pressor BP responsivity data collected by Hines and Brown in the 1930s (Hines, 1937a; Hines, 1937b). Findings indicated that 71% of subjects classified as hyperreactive in childhood (6–19 years of age) had developed EH in adulthood. Using a sample of borderline hypertensive adolescents, Falkner, Kushner, Onesti, and Angelakos (1981) observed that those who developed EH 5 years later had the greatest BP responsivity to a psychological stressor at initial screening, and also had a family history of EH. With some exceptions (Eiff, Gogolin, Jacobs, & Neus, 1985; Hofman & Valkenburg, 1983; Visser, Grobbee, & Hofman, 1987), a rather consistent body of studies has accumulated which indicates that CVR in youth is predictive of future CV functioning in youth. These studies utilized a variety of stressors (e.g., cold pressor, dynamic exercise, mental arithmetic, star tracing, video game) and found BP responsivity to be predictive of resting BP levels 1–6 years later. These findings remained after accounting for contributions of various BP risk factors such as age, initial resting BP levels, and adiposity (Alpert, Murphy, & Treiber, 1994; Mahoney et al., 1988; Matthews, Woodall, & Stoney, 1990; Murphy, 1992; Newman, McGarvey, & Steele, 1999; Parker et al., 1987; Treiber, Del Rosario, Davis, Gutlin, & Strong, 1997; Treiber et al., 1994; Treiber, Musante, Kapuku, Davis, Litaker, & Davis, 2001; Treiber, Turner, Davis, Thompson, Levy, & Strong, 1996). For example, Murphy and colleagues consistently observed that exaggerated BP responses to a video game challenge were predictive of resting BP 1–4 years later in a sample of white and African American youth initially evaluated in the third grade (Murphy, Alpert, & Walker, 1992; Murphy et al., 1991; Murphy et al., 1994). Matthews, Woodall, and Allen (1993) found BP increases to mental arithmetic were predictive of resting BP 6 years later in a group of white middle-class youth initially 6–12 years old.

Findings from several recent longitudinal studies have corroborated and extended earlier findings of CVR prediction studies by including prediction of the underlying hemodynamic regulators of BP control (i.e., TPR, CO). Two studies using the same cohort of white and African American 6–7 year-olds found BP responses to stressors (forehead cold, exercise, postural change) to be predictive of resting BP 1 and 22 years later even after controlling for baseline BP levels and significant baseline anthropometric and demographic characteristics (Malpass, Treiber, Turner, Davis, Thompson, Levy, & Strong, 1997; Treiber et al., 1996). Another ongoing cohort study involving youth (initial average age 11.5 years) with family histories of EH found that after controlling for the significant contributions of traditional risk factors including gender, ethnicity, anthropometrics (e.g., height, weight, adiposity) and initial baseline CV data, resting systolic and diastolic BP were predicted by respective BP stress responses to video game challenge, postural change, and forehead cold at 1- and 5-year follow-ups (Treiber, Davis, Thompson, Levy, & Strong, 1997; Treiber et al., 1994). Importantly, although stress responses were not predictive of subsequent TPR at the 1-year follow-up, by the 5-year follow-up, resting TPR was predicted by TPR video game responsivity, after accounting for the significant contributions of weight and gender (males > females). Collectively, these findings suggest that during early pubertal transition, prediction of vasoconstrictive function is problematic.

However, by late adolescence, vasoconstrictive responsivity to active coping challenges in childhood are predictive of vasoconstrictive functioning.

Prediction of Ventricular Remodeling

Left ventricular hypertrophy is an important predictor of cardiovascular morbidity (e.g., arrhythmia, congestive heart failure, MI) and all cause mortality (Koren et al., 1991; Levy, 1991; Mensah, Liao, & Cooper, 1995). Echocardiographic studies involving children and adolescents, many of which involved hypertensives or those with elevated resting pressures, have collectively shown increased LVM to be positively related to resting BP, age, gender (boys > girls), physical inactivity, and various indices of body habitus including height, weight, body surface area, and adiposity (Burke, Arcilla, Culpepper, Webber, Chiang, & Berenson, 1987; Goble, Mosteller, Moskowitz, & Schieken, 1992; Radice, Alli, Avanzini, Di Tullio, Mariotti, Taioli, Zussino, & Folli, 1986; Schieken, Clarke, & Lauer, 1981; Urbina, Gidding, Bao, Pickoff, Berdusis, & Berenson, 1995; Zahka, Neill, Kidd, Cutilletta, & Cutilletta, 1981).

Relatively few cross-sectional studies have been conducted that involved CVR to laboratory stressors as possible correlates of increased LVM. Daniels, Meyer, and Loggie (1990) noted that body size, dietary sodium intake, gender (boys > girls), and peak systolic pressure responses to dynamic exercise were all significant independent correlates of LVM indexed by height in a sample of hypertensive 6–23 year-olds. Using a sample of prepubertal 6–12 year-old whites, Janz, Burns, and Mahoney (1995) examined correlates of LVM after adjusting for fat-free mass and adiposity. Although a number of parameters were significant at the univariate level, including resting BP, measures of physical fitness (peak VO_2, peak work and grip strength), and indices of physical activity (global ratings and television viewing time), multiple regression results revealed that only peak systolic BP responses to exercise remained as a significant independent correlate. Treiber, McCaffrey, Pflieger, Raunikar, Strong, and Davis (1993) also used multiple regression analyses and observed that in a sample of 6–18 year-olds with a positive family history of EH, that TPR responsivity to forehead cold stimulation was a significant determinant of $LVM/height^{2.7}$, after accounting for other significant correlates which included adiposity, gender (boys > girls), age, and resting systolic BP.

Only a few prospective LVM studies that included measures of CVR to stress have been conducted with youth. Mahoney et al. (1988) conducted a 3–4-year prospective study and found that after accounting for the contributions of initial LVM, the only other parameter to enter the statistical model as an independent contributor was peak diastolic BP response to dynamic exercise (bicycle ergometry). Recently, Murdison et al. (1998) examined predictors of LVM/height$^{2.7}$ from data collected an average of 2.6 years earlier in a sample of white and African American normotensive youth with family histories of EH (mean age 12.9 ± 2.9 years at initial visit). Using multiple regression analyses, follow-up LVM/height$^{2.7}$ was predicted by the initial LVM/height$^{2.7}$, weight, ethnicity (African Americans > whites) and an aggregate index of BP responsivity to a battery of laboratory stressors (i.e., parent child conflict discussion, social stressor interview, video game challenge, and postural change). Further, youth classified as having LVH based upon gender- and age-specific norms (Daniels, Meyer, Liang, and Bove, 1988) at follow-up, were found to be differentiated at the initial evaluation on several parameters including having greater height, weight, adiposity, higher resting BP and greater aggregated BP responsivity to laboratory stressors (Murdison et al., 1998). Papavassiliou, Treiber, Strong, Malpass, and Davis (1996) examined the predictors of LVM an average of 3.6 years after an initial evaluation in a sample of white and African American children (mean age 7.9 ± 0.7 years at initial evaluation). Using parameters significant at the univariate level, multiple regression analyses indicated that initial weight, height, and CO responsivity to postural change and treadmill exercise were significant predictors of LVM. Similar analyses were conducted predicting LVM indexed by height$^{2.7}$ which indicated that initial adiposity as well as CO and systolic BP responsivity to postural change were significant predictors of future LVM/height$^{2.7}$.

Recently, Kapuku, Treiber, Davis, Harshfield, Cook, and Mensah (1999) examined predictors of future LVM in a cohort of 71 EA and 75 AA normotensive adolescents. Subjects were initially an average of 14.2–1.8 years of age and evaluated on two occasions separated by an average of 2.3 years. SBP reactivity to a virtual reality car driving simulation was a significant independent predictor of LVM/body surface area at follow-up even after adjustment for the significant contributions of initial LVM/body surface area, weight, gender (males > females), and baseline resting total peripheral resistance. However, this association was not consistent when LVM was indexed by height$^{2.7}$. Although SBP reactivity was significantly related to follow-up LVM/height$^{2.7}$ at the univariate level, it did not add significantly to a multiple regression model in which initial LVM/height$^{2.7}$, BMI, gender, and supine resting total peripheral resistance were already included.

Examinations of components of LV geometry were also conducted by Papavassiliou et al. (1996). Increased relative wall thickness was predicted by ethnicity (African Americans > whites), adiposity, and systolic pressure responsivity to postural change. Left ventricular internal diameter was predicted by baseline height and diastolic pressure responsivity to forehead cold stimulation. To our knowledge, this is the first study to examine the predictors of these components of LV geometry in youth. These findings indicate that, in youth with family histories of EH, African Americans may exhibit early indications of concentric remodeling prior to development of elevated BP, and that this is related in part to exaggerated CVR to stress. Given that African Americans frequently exhibit greater relative wall thickness, have a higher prevalence of hypertension, and have a greater likelihood of developing concentric hypertrophy than whites as adults, these findings are particularly important (Hinderliter, Light, & Willis, 1992). Collectively, these findings indicate that CVR to stress in childhood appears to be a significant contributor to concurrent, and, more importantly, to future increases in LVM after accounting for contributions of standard risk factors.

Prediction of Vascular Remodeling

As predicted in Figure 5.1 under ARMs I & II, vascular smooth muscle hypertrophy, along with continued lipid accumulations leading to fatty streaks and eventually lesions, results in decreased arterial elasticity (Hollander, Madoff, Paddock, & Kirkpatrick, 1976; Wolinsky, Goldfischer, Daly, Kasak, & Coltoff-Schiller, 1975). Riley, Freedman, Higgs, Barnes, Zinkgraf, and Berenson (1986) examined carotid artery wall elasticity in a sample of the Bogalusa Heart Study cohort at 10–17 years of age. Findings indicated that several markers of response potential were related to decreased elasticity. An ethnic difference was observed in which African American youth exhibited lower elasticity compared to whites. Males were also found to have lower elasticity than females. Finally, after controlling for ethnicity, gender and age, decreased elasticity was still associated with a positive family history of MI. Given that decreased carotid elasticity has been associated with coronary artery lesions in adults (Crouse III, Kahl, Schez, Toole, & McKinney, 1984; Holme, Enger, Helgeland, Hjermann, Leren, Lund-Larsen, Solberg, & Strong, 1981), evaluation of possible associations between CVR and changes in superficial arterial wall elasticity prior to overt manifestation of CVD is warranted.

The third arm of the model portrays another functional manifestation of vascular remodeling that occurs quite early in the pathogenesis of CVD, namely decreased endothelium dependent arterial dilation (EDAD) in response to reactive hyperemia (Celermajer, Sorensen, Barley, Jeffrey, Carter, & Deanfield, 1994; Celermajer, Sorensen, Bull, Robinson, & Deanfield, 1994; Celermajer et al., 1993; Celermajer et al., 1992). Recent studies evaluating EDAD using high resolution ultrasound have shown that adults with various manifestations of CVD, including EH and atherosclerosis, and youth with familial hypercholesterolemia exhibited less vasodilation of the femoral or brachial arteries in response to reactive hyperemia compared to healthy cohorts (Anderson, Uehata, Gerhard, Meredith, Knab, Delagrange, Lieberman, Ganz, Creager, Yeung, & Selwyn, 1995; Celermajer et al., 1992; Sorensen, Celermajer, Georgakopoulos, Hatcher, Betteridge, & Deanfield, 1994). Smoking, family history of premature CVD, elevated cholesterol, increased resting BP levels, and male gender have all been associated with decreased flow-mediated vasodilation in a sample of 5–73-year-olds (mean age = 36 years) (Celermajer, Sorensen, Bull, Robinson, & Deanfield, 1994).

To our knowledge, only one published study has evaluated the relationships between CVR to laboratory stressors with EDAD. Treiber et al. (1997) evaluated EDAD of the superficial femoral artery in response to 5 min of blood flow occlusion using a protocol established by Celermajer et al. (1992). In a sample of 11–13-year-olds who varied in their family history of premature MI, decreased EDAD was associated with increased systolic BP responsivity to all three stressors administered (i.e., forehead cold, postural change, supine cycle ergometry), increased adiposity, including sum of skinfold thickness and percent fat via dual energy x-ray absorptiometry, and decreased cardiovascular fitness. No differences in EDAD were observed by gender, ethnicity, or family history of premature MI. Multiple regression analyses indicated that an index of CV fitness and systolic BP responsivity to supine exercise were the only significant independent correlates of EDAD. Interestingly, CV fitness was significantly related to all of the other variables which had been related to EDAD at the univariate level. These findings are provocative, but cross validation with larger sample sizes and more diverse types of subjects is required. If these findings are replicated, the importance of aerobic fitness and physical training programs in youth with regard to potential improvements upon various components of CV health, such as body fatness, resting BP, HR, lipids/lipoprotein profiles and potential endothelial function, would be supported (Gutin, Cucuzzo, Islam, Smith, Moffatt, & Pargman, 1995; Murphy, 1992; Van Doornen & De Geus, 1989).

Endothelial dysfunction has been found to be a relatively early event in the atherogenesis of CVD. Figure 1 illustrates how the damage to the endothelium results in a decreased ability to release endothelium-derived relaxing factors in response to increased flow (Meredith, Yeung, & Weidinger, 1993; Zeiher, Drexler, Wollschlager, & Just, 1991). One aspect of this damage involves the potentially increased production of ET-1, the most potent vasoconstrictive peptide produced in man (Davies et al., 1995; Lemne, Lundeberg, Theodorsson, & de Faire, 1994; Luscher & Vanhoutte, 1990). Adults studies have shown that resting plasma ET-1 levels vary by ethnicity, gender, and CVD status. Although not entirely consistent, among adults with EH, African Americans have been found to have higher baseline level of ET-1 than whites (Ergul, Parish, Puett, & Ergul, 1996; Evans, Phillips, Singh, Bauman, & Gulati, 1996). Several adult studies involving normotensives with a positive family history of EH or individuals with borderline or established EH demonstrate that these individuals have higher basal levels of ET-1 compared to normotensive controls (Lemne et al., 1994). Healthy men have been found to have higher levels of ET-1 than healthy women (Polderman, Steouwer, van Kamp, Dekker, Verheugt, & Gooren, 1993). To our knowledge, only two studies have been conducted in adults which examined the relationship between CVR and ET-1 levels. In both, findings indicated that ET-1 increased significantly in response to psychological stressors (Fyhrquist, Saijonmaa, Metsarinne, Tikkanen, Rosenlof, & Tikkanen, 1990; Noll, Wenzel, Schneider, Oesch, Binggeli, Shaw, Weidmann, & Luscher, 1996).

Finally, a study was recently conducted in our laboratory with a sample of adolescent white and African American males with positive family histories of EH (Treiber, Jackson, Davis, Pollock, Kapuku, Mensah, & Pollock, 2000). ET-1 levels were evaluated at rest and in response to a video game challenge and cold pressor stimulation. The findings indicated that the African Americans had higher levels of ET-1 and TPR immediately after catheter insertion and at every time point throughout the protocol. African Americans also showed greater increases in ET-1 to both stressors along with forehead cold along with the expected significantly greater increases in TPR responsivity. Although these findings are promising, replication with larger sample sizes is required.

CLINICAL CARE IMPLICATIONS

While the clinical care implications have been noted in passing in several places throughout this chapter, it is worth bringing them together at this point. CVD remains the leading cause of death of American adults almost 1 million per year die from the various forms of CVD. We now know that the origins of CVD occur at a much earlier age than once thought, with atherogenesis commencing in the childhood years. Identification of the disease process at an early stage offers the chance for successful preventive interventions, which are beneficial for the individual and also for society, since the cost of prevention is likely to be much less than the cost of treatment. Given the present levels of CVD in adults, the potential health care costs for future generations are considerable.

Research has enabled the identification of preclinical markers of future CVD. These markers are changes in CV structure and/or function that are not in themselves classified as clinical symptoms but which portend such symptoms if the etiologic process is not arrested. The current literature suggests that excessive responsivity to stress might be a useful preclinical marker. If further research supports this notion, psychological and/or physical stress testing might contribute useful information (along with items such as elevated resting BP, and changes in cardiac morphology) when deciding whether intervention is warranted.

The significance of this work is particularly relevant for pediatric populations. The sooner primary intervention can be commenced with at risk individuals, the greater the chances of ameliorating disease progression. The studies reviewed in this chapter suggest both that preclinical markers of CVD can be identified in youths, and that these markers are likely to be convincingly shown to be predictive of CVD. Collectively, these findings point to the need for development of effective CVD primary prevention approaches in youth. For example, a variety of nonpharmacologic approaches have been used in efforts to lower BP in youth. Several recent reviews have indicated that electrolyte control/supplementation, diet and/or physical exercise interventions over 1 month–3 year intervals have met with mixed results, with most studies finding minimal to no effect upon resting BP in normotensive youth (Alpert, Murphy, & Treiber, 1994; Resnicow, 1993). Given the inconsistency in electrolyte control/supplementation, diet and/or exercise interventions upon BP control and the potential role of psychosocial stress in the development of EH, stress reduction approaches may prove to be more beneficial in reduction of BP in youth. However, to date, results from only one stress reduction intervention in youth have been published. Ewart, Harris, Iwata, Coates, Bullock, and Simon (1987) evaluated the efficacy of progressive muscle relaxation training in predominantly White adolescents with BP between the eighty-fifth and ninety-fifth percentiles for age. Progressive muscle relaxation instruction provided in class for academic credit for 12 weeks was compared to a traditional no contact control condition. Progressive muscle relaxation reduced SBP relative to the controls at posttreatment (−7.2 vs −1.9 mmHg). However, at a 16-week follow-up there were no longer significant differences between the two groups in resting SBP.

An 8-week randomized controlled pilot study was recently conducted which examined the effects of stress reduction on hemodynamic function in 16 adolescents with high normal BP (Barnes, Treiber, Davis, & Strong, 1998). Blood pressure screenings on a random sample of 100 youth at a local high school identified 16 adolescents (15 African Americans, 1 white; ages 15–18 years) with resting SBP in the eighty-fifth and ninety-fifth percentile range on 3 consecutive occasions. A pretreatment evaluation was conducted of CV functioning at rest and during a battery of 3 laboratory stressors. Subjects were then randomly assigned to either a Transcendental Meditation (TM) group (n = 8) or a health education control (CTL, n = 8). After receiving the formal 5-session course in TM by a certified instructor, the TM group engaged in 15 min TM sessions during the school lunch break and at home each day for 8 weeks. The CTL group was given information on lowering BP through weight loss (if needed), improved diet (reducing fat and sodium and increasing fruit and vegetable intake) and increasing physical activity. In terms of intervention effects, from pre- to posttreatment, the TM group exhibited greater increases in resting stroke volume ($p < .05$), and trends for greater decreases in resting SBP and TPR ($ps < .12$) compared to the control group. The TM group exhibited decreased SBP reactivity to a virtual reality car driving stressor and decreased CO reactivity to a social stressor interview compared to the control group ($ps < .05$). Given the small sample size, these results are not definitive, but the pattern of findings are encouraging and point out the need for further evaluation of the impact of behavioral stress reduction approaches upon preclinical manifestation of CVD in at risk youth.

SUMMARY

This chapter has presented a biobehavioral model of CVR as a possible mechanism leading to overt manifestation of CVD via ventricular and vascular remodeling. The literature in youth to date supporting this model was discussed. As noted earlier, this model is not meant to include all possible mechanistic pathways leading to CVD (e.g., familial hypercholesterolemia, smoking, diet, renin-angiotensin system, sodium sensitivity, etc. (Schneiderman & Skyler, 1996). Also, within this model not all possible pathways are delineated. For example, fatty streaks may have a direct impact upon decreased EDAD prior to development of plaque formation and more advanced forms of atherosclerosis. Furthermore, there may be perturbations in the model, particularly during periods of rapid development (e.g., puberty), some of which may partially explain lack of consistency in the results from various CVR studies involving wide age ranges of youth. The pathways explicated in the model were chosen for inclusion based upon their support by the vast majority of CVR studies in youth. Thus, this model may be helpful in guiding future research examining the relationship between CVR and preclinical manifestations of CVD in youth.

The recent advances in vascular biology and noninvasive CV technology now permit the examination of underlying mechanisms which will potentially provide linkages between CVR early in life to progressive changes in preclinical markers of CVD leading to overt endpoints. While the data so far are encouraging, further studies are needed to determine whether the proposed model follows the progression predicted leading to overt CVD endpoints. In the meantime, the data presented support an increased attention to the development of primary prevention stress reduction programs which will decrease CVR and hopefully alter the progressive development of CVD related risk factors in at risk youth.

REFERENCES

Akinkubge, O. O. (1985). World epidemiology of hypertension in blacks. In W. D. Hall, E. Saunders, & N. B. Shulman (Eds.), *Hypertension in blacks: Epidemiology, pathophysiology and treatment* (pp. 3–16). Chicago: Yearbook Publishers.

Allen, M. T., & Matthews, K. A. (1997). Hemodynamic responses to laboratory stressors in children and adolescents: The influences of age, race, and gender. *Psychophysiology, 34*(3), 329–339.

Alpert, B. S., Dover, E. V., Booker, D. L., Martin, A. M., & Strong, W. B. (1981). Blood pressure response to dynamic exercise in healthy children—black vs white. *Journal of Pediatrics, 99,* 556–560.

Alpert, B. S., Murphy, J. K., & Christman, J. V. (1986). Does fitness protect against excessive heart rate reactivity to psychologic stress? *Pediatric Research, 20,* 167A.

Alpert, B. S., Murphy, J. K., & Treiber, F. A. (1994). Essential hypertension: Approaches to prevention in children. *Medical Exercise Nutrition of Health, 3,* 296–307.

Alpert, B. S., & Wilson, D. K. (1992). Stress reactivity in childhood and adolescence. In J. R. Turner, A. Sherwood, & K. C. Light (Eds.), *Individual differences in cardiovascular response to stress* (pp. 187–201). New York: Plenum.

American Heart Association. (2000). *Heart and Stroke Facts: 2001 Statistical Supplement.* Dallas, Texas.

Anderson, N. B., McNeilly, M., & Myers, H. (1991). Autonomic reactivity and hypertension in blacks: A review and proposed model. *Ethnicity and Disease, 1,* 154–170.

Anderson, T. J., Uehata, A., Gerhard, M. D., Meredith, I. T., Knab, S., Delagrange, D., Lieberman, E. H., Ganz, P., Creager, M. A., Yeung, A. C., & Selwyn, A. P. (1995). Close relation of endothelial function in the human coronary and peripheral circulations. *Journal of the American College of Cardiology, 26,* 1235–1241.

Andrawis, N. S., Wang, E., & Abernethy, D. R. (1996). Endothelin-1 induces an increase in total protein synthesis and expression of the smooth muscle alpha-actin gene in vascular smooth musce cells. *Life Sciences, 59,* 523–528.

Arbeit, M. L., Johnson, C. C., & Mot, D. S. (1992). The heart smart cardiovascular school health promotion Behavior correlates of risk factor changes. *Preventive Medicine, 21,* 18–32.

Arensman, F. W., Treiber, F. A., Gruber, M. P., & Strong, W. B. (1989). Exercise-induced differences in cardiac output, blood pressure and systemic vascular resistance in a healthy biracial population of ten-year-old boys. *American Journal of Diseases of Children, 143,* 212–216.

Barnes, V. A., Treiber, F. A., Davis, H., & Strong, W. B. (1998). *Effects of transcendental meditation on cardiovascular reactivity in adolescents with high normal blood pressure.* Presentation, American Psychosomatic Society.

Barnett, P. H., Hines, Jr., E. A., Schirger, A., & Gage, R. P. (1963). Blood pressure and vascular reactivity to the cold pressor test: Restudy of 207 subjects 27 years later. *Journal of the American Medical Association, 183,* 845–848.

Berenson, G. S. (1986). *Causation of cardiovascular risk factors in children: Perspectives on cardiovascular risk in early life.* New York: Raven Press.

Berenson, G. S., McMahan, C., Voors, A. W., Webber, L., Srinivasan, S. R., Frank, G. C., Foster, T. A., & Blonde, C. V. (1980). *Cardiovascular risk factors in children: The early natural history of atherosclerosis and essential hypertension.* New York: Oxford University Press.

Berenson, G. S., Wattigney, W. A., Tracy, R. E., Newman, W. P., Srinivasan, S. R., Webber, L. S., Dalferes, E. R., Jr., & Strong, J. P. (1992). Atherosclerosis of the aorta and coronary arteries and cardiovascular risk factors in persons aged 6 to 30 years and studied at necropsy (The Bogalusa Heart Study). *American Journal of Cardiology, 70,* 851–858.

Burke, G. L., Arcilla, R. A., Culpepper, W. S., Webber, L. S., Chiang, Y., & Berenson, G. S. (1987). Blood pressure and echocardiographic measures in children: The Bogalusa Heart Study. *Circulation, 75,* 106–114.

Burt, V. L., Whelton, P., Roccella, E. J., Brown, C., Cutler, J. A., Higgins, M., Horan, M. J., & Labarthe, D. (1995). Prevalence of hypertension in the U.S. adult population Results from the Third National Health and Nutrition Examination Survey, 1988–1991. *Hypertension, 25,* 305–313.

Casale, P. N., Devereux, R. B., Milner, M., Zullo, G., Harshfield, G. A., Pickering, G. W., & Laragh, J. H. (1986). Value of echocardiographic measurement of left ventricular mass in predicting cardiovascular morbid events in hypertensive men. *Annals of Internal Medicine, 105,* 173–178.

Celermajer, D. S., Sorensen, K. E., Barley, J., Jeffrey, S., Carter, N., & Deanfield, J. (1994). Angiotensin-converting enzyme genotype is not associated with endothelial dysfunction in subjects without other coronary risk factors. *Atherosclerosis, 111,* 121–126.

Celermajer, D. S., Sorensen, K. E., Bull, C., Robinson, J., & Deanfield, J. E. (1994). Endothelium-dependent dilation in the systemic arteries of asymptomatic subjects relates to coronary risk factors and their interaction. *Journal of the American College of Cardiology, 24,* 1468–1474.

Celermajer, D. S., Sorensen, K. E., Georgakopoulos, D., Bull, C., Thomas, O., Robinson, J., & Deanfield, J. E. (1993). Cigarette smoking is associated with dose-related and potentially reversible impairment of endothelium-dependent dilation in healthy young adults. *Circulation, 88,* 2149–2155.

Celermajer, D. S., Sorensen, K. E., Gooch, V. M., Spiegelhalter, D. J., Miller, O. I., Sullivan, I. D., Lloyd, J. K., & Vernfield, J. E. (1992). Non-invasive detection of endothelial dysfunction in children and adults at risk of atherosclerosis. *Lancet, 340,* 1111–1115.

Coates, T. J., Parker, F. C., & Kolodner, K. (1982). Stress and heart disease: Does blood pressure reactivity offer a link? In T. J. Coates & A. C. Peterson (Eds.), *Promoting adolescent health* (pp. 305–321). New York: Academic.

Crouse, III, J., Kahl, F., Schez, H., Toole, J., & McKinney, W. (1984). Is carotid artery atherosclerosis an indicator of coronary artery disease? *Circulation, 70,* 11–66.

Daniels, S. D., Meyer, R. A., & Loggie, J. M. H. (1990). Determinants of cardiac involvement in children and adolescents with essential hypertension. *Circulation, 82,* 1243–1248.

Daniels, S. R., Meyer, R. A., Liang, Y., & Bove, K. E. (1988). Echocardiographically determined left ventricular mass index in normal children, adolescents and young adults. *Journal of the American College of Cardiology, 12,* 703–708.

Davies, P. F., Barbee, K. A., Lal, R., Robotewskyj, A., & Griem, M. L. (1995). Hemodynamics and atherogenesis: Endothelial surface dynamics in flow signal transduction. In F. Numano & R. W. Wissler (Eds.), *Atherosclerosis III: Recent advances in atherosclerosis research* (pp. 86–103). New York: Annals of the New York Academy of Sciences.

Del Rosario, J. D., Treiber, F. A., Harshfield, G. A., Davis, H. C., & Strong, W. B. (1998). Predictors of future ambulatory blood pressure in youth. *Journal of Pediatrics, 132,* 693–698.

Devereux, R., de Simone, G., Koren, M., Roman, M., & Laragh, J. (1991). Left ventricular mass as a predictor of development of hypertension. *American Journal of Hypertension, 4,* 603–607.

Devereux, R. B., & Alderman, M. H. (1993). Role of preclinical cardiovascular disease in the evolution from risk factor exposure to development of morbid events. *Circulation, 88,* 1444–1455.

Devereux, R. B., Koren, M. J., de Simone, G., Roman, M. J., & Laragh, J. H. (1992). Left ventricular mass as a measure of preclinical hypertensive disease. *American Journal of Hypertension, 5,* 175–181.

Dysart, J. M., Treiber, F. A., Pflieger, K., Davis, H., & Strong, W. (1994). Ethnic differences in the myocardial and vascular reactivity to stress in normotensive girls. *American Journal of Hypertension, 7,* 15–22.

Eiff, A. W., Gogolin, E., Jacobs, V., & Neus, H. (1985). Heart rate reactivity under mental stress as a predictor of blood pressure development in children. *Journal of Hypertension, 3,* 89–91.

Ergul, S., Parish, D. C., Puett, D., & Ergul, A. (1996). Racial differences in plasma endothelin-1 concentrations in individuals with essential hypertension [published erratum appears in *Hypertension 1997 Mar. 29*(3), 912]. *Hypertension, 28,* 652–655.

Evans, R. R., Phillips, B. G., Singh, G., Bauman, J. L., & Gulati, A. (1996). Racial and gender differences in endothelin-1. *American Journal of Cardiology, 78,* 486–488.

Ewart, C. K., Harris, W. L., Iwata, M. M., Coates, T. J., Bullock, R., & Simon, B. (1987). Feasibility and effectiveness of school-based relaxation in lowering blood pressure. *Health Psychology, 6,* 399–416.

Ewart, C. K., & Kolodner, K. B. (1993). Predicting ambulatory blood pressure during school: Effectiveness of social and nonsocial reactivity tasks in black and white adolescents. *Psychophysiology, 30,* 30–38.

Falkner, B., & Kushner, H. (1989). Race differences in stress-induced reactivity in young adults. *Health Psychology, 8,* 613–627.

Falkner, B., Kushner, H., Onesti, G., & Angelakos, E. T. (1981). Cardiovascular characteristics in adolescents who develop essential hypertension. *Hypertension, 3,* 521–527.

Fillingim, R. B., & Blumenthal, J. A. (1992). Does aerobic exercise reduce stress responses? In J. R. Turner, A. Sherwood, & K. C. Light (Eds.), *Individual differences in cardiovascular response to stress* (pp. 203–217). New York: Plenum.

Folkow, B. (1990). The structural factor in hypertension. In J. H. Laragh & S. M. Brenner (Eds.), *Hypertension: Pathophysiology, diagnosis and management* (pp. 5–58). New York: Raven Press, Ltd.

Folkow, B. (1990). "Structural Factor" in primary and secondary hypertension. *Hypertension, 16,* 89–101.

Folkow, B., Grimby, G., & Thulesius, O. (1958). Adaptive structural changes of the vascular walls in hypertension and their relation to the control of the peripheral resistance. *Acta Physiologica Scandinavica, 44,* 255–272.

Fredrikson, M., & Matthews, K. A. (1990). Cardiovascular responses to behavioral stress and hypertension: A meta-analytic review. *Annals of Behavioral Medicine, 12,* 30–39.

Fuster, V., Badimon, L., Badimon, J. J., & Chesebro, J. H. (1992). The pathogenesis of coronary artery disease and the acute coronary syndromes. *New England Journal of Medicine, 326,* 310–318.

Fyhrquist, F., Saijonmaa, O., Metsarinne, K., Tikkanen, I., Rosenlof, K., & Tikkanen, T. (1990). Raised plasma endothelin-1 concentration following cold pressor test. *Biochemical and Biophysical Research Communications, 169,* 217–221.

Genest, J., Koiw, E., & Kuchel, O. (1977). *Hypertension—Physiopathology and treatment.* New York: McGraw-Hill.

Gillum, R. F. (1991). Cardiovascular disease in the United States: An epidemiologic overview. In E. Saunders (Ed.), *Cardiovascular diseases in blacks* (Vol. 21, pp. 3–16). New York: F. A. Davis Company.

Gimbrone, M. A., Cybulsky, M. I., Kume, N., Collins, T., & Resnick, N. (1995). Vascular endothelium: An integrator of pathophysiological stimuli in atherogenesis. *Atherosclerosis III: Recent advances in atherosclerosis research* (Vol. 748, pp. 122–132). New York: Annals of the New York Academy of Sciences.

Giordani, B., Manuck, S., & Farmer, J. (1981). Stability of behaviorally-induced heart rate changes in children after one week. *Child Development, 52,* 533–537.

Girdler, S. S., Turner, J. R., Sherwood, A., & Light, K. C. (1990). Sex differences in blood pressure control during a variety of behavioral stressors. *Psychosomatic Medicine, 52,* 571–591.

Goble, M. M., Mosteller, M., Moskowitz, W. B., & Schieken, R. M. (1992). Sex differences in the determinants of left ventricular mass in childhood: The Medical College of Virginia Twin Study. *Circulation, 85,* 1661–1665.

Gutin, B., Cucuzzo, N., Islam, S., Smith, C., Moffatt, R., & Pargman, D. (1995). Physical training improves body composition of black obese 7 to 11 year old girls. *Obesity Research, 3,* 305–312.

Gutin, B., Manos, T., Manghram, E., Thompson, W., & Treiber, F. (1993). Physical training, fatness and reactive blood pressure in boys. *Pediatric Exercise Science, 5,* 425.

Hagberg, J. M., Goldring, D., Health, G. W., Ehsani, A. A., Hernandez, A., & Holloszy, J. O. (1984). Effect of exercise training on plasma catecholamines and haemodynamics of adolescent hypertensive during rest, submaximal exercise and orthostatic stress. *Clinical Physiology, 4,* 117–124.

Harshfield, G. A., Alpert, B. S., Willey, E. S., Somes, G. W., Murphy, J. K., & Dupaul, L. M. (1989). Race and gender influence ambulatory blood pressure patterns of adolescents. *Hypertension, 14,* 598–603.

Harshfield, G. A., Dupaul, L. M., Alpert, B. S., Christman, J. V., Willey, E. S., Murphy, J. K., & Somes, G. W. (1990). Aerobic fitness and the diurnal rhythm of blood pressure in adolescents. *Hypertension, 15,* 810–814.

Hinderliter, A. L., Light, K. C., & Willis, P. W. (1992). Racial differences in left ventricular structure in healthy young adults. *American Journal of Cardiology, 69,* 1196–1199.

Hines, E. A. (1937a). The hereditary factor in essential hypertension. *Annals of Internal Medicine, 11,* 593–601.

Hines, E. A. (1937b). Reaction of the blood pressure of 400 school children to a standard stimulus. *Journal of the American Medical Association, 108,* 1249–1250.

Hofman, A., & Valkenburg, H. A. (1983). Determinants of change in blood pressure during childhood. *American Journal of Epidemiology, 117,* 735–743.

Hollander, W., Madoff, I., Paddock, J., & Kirkpatrick, B. (1976). Aggravation of atherosclerosis by hypertension in a subhuman primate model with coarctation of the aorta. *Circulation Research, 38,* 63–72.

Holme, I., Enger, S. C., Helgeland, A., Hjermann, I., Leren, P., Lund-Larsen, P. G., Solberg, L. A., & Strong, J. P. (1981). Risk factors and raised atherosclerotic lesions in coronary and cerebral arteries. Statistical analysis from the Oslo study. *Arteriosclerosis, 1,* 250–256.

Hypertension Detection and Follow-up Program Cooperative Group. (1984). Five-year findings of the Hypertension Detection and Follow-up Programs Mortality by race-sex and blood pressure level—A further analysis. *Journal of Community Health,* *9,* 314–317.

Ichikawa, K. I., Hidai, C., Okuda, C., Kimata, S. I., Matsuoka, R., Hosoda, S., Quertermous, T., & Kawana, M. (1996). Endogenous endothelin-1 mediates cardiac hypertrophy and switching of myosin heavy chain gene expression in rat ventricular myocardium. *Journal of the American College of Cardiology, 27,* 1286–1291.

James, S. A., Harinett, S. A., & Kalsbeek, W. D. (1983). John Henryism and blood pressure differences among black men. *Journal of Behavioral Medicine, 6,* 259–278.

Janz, K. F., Burns, T. L., & Mahoney, L. T. (1995). Predictors of left ventricular mass and resting blood pressure in children: The Muscatine Study. *Medicine and Science in Sports and Exercise, 27,* 818–825.

Jiang, W., Babyak, M., Krantz, D. S., Waugh, R. A., Coleman, R. E., Hanson, M. M., Fied, D. J., McNulty, S., Morris, J. J., O'Connor, C. M., & Blumenthal, J. A. (1996). Mental-stress induced myocardial-ischemia and cardiac events. *Journal of the American Medical Association, 275,* 1651–1656.

Johnson, E. H., Schork, N. J., & Spielberger, C. D. (1987). Emotional and familial determinants of elevated blood pressure in black and white adolescent females. *Journal of Psychosomatic Research, 31,* 731–741.

Johnson, E. H., Spielberger, C. D., Worden, T. J., & Jacobs, G. A. (1987). Emotional and familial determinants of elevated blood pressure in black and white adolescent males. *Journal of Psychosomatic Research, 31,* 287–300.

Kamarck, T. W., Jennings, J. R., Debski, T. T., Glickman-Weiss, E., Johnson, P. S., Eddy, M. J., & Manuck, S. B. (1992). Reliable measures of behaviorally-evoked cardiovascular reactivity from a PC-based test battery: Results from student and community samples. *Psychophysiology, 29,* 17–28.

Kamarck, T. W., Jennings, J. R., Stewart, C. J., & Eddy, M. J. (1993). Reliable responses to a cardiovascular reactivity protocol: A replication study in a biracial female sample. *Psychophysiology, 30,* 627–634.

Kapuku, G., Treiber, F. A., Davis, H. C., Harshfield, G. A., Cook, B. B., & Mensah, G. A. (1999). Hemodynamic function at rest, during acute stress, and in the field: Predictors of cardiac structure and function 2 years later in youth. *Hypertension, 34,* 1026–1031.

Koren, M. J., Devereux, R. B., Casale, P. N., Savage, D. D., & Laragh, J. H. (1991). Relation of left ventricular mass and geometry to morbidity and mortality in uncomplicated essential hypertension. *Annals of Internal Medicine, 114,* 345–352.

Krantz, D. S., & Manuck, S. B. (1984). Acute psychophysiologic reactivity and risk of cardiovascular disease: A review and methodologic critique. *Psychological Bulletin, 96,* 435–464.

Langewitz, W., Ruddel, H., Schachinger, H., & Schmieder, R. (1989). Standardized stress testing in the cardiovascular laboratory: Has it any bearing on ambulatory blood pressure values? *Journal of Hypertension, 7,* 41–48.

Lemne, C. E., Lundeberg, T., Theodorsson, E., & de Faire, U. (1994). Increased basal concentrations of plasma endothelin in borderline hypertension. *Journal of Hypertension, 12,* 1069–1074.

Levy, D. (1991). Clinical significance of left ventricular hypertrophy: Insights from the Framingham Study. *Journal of Cardiovascular Pharmacology, 17,* 1–6.

Light, K. C. (1989). Constitutional factors relating to differences in cardiovascular response. In N. Schneiderman, S. M. Weiss, & P. G. Kaufman (Eds.), *Handbook of research methods in cardiovascular behavioral medicine* (pp. 413–431). New York: Plenum Press.

Light, K. C., Turner, J. R., Hinderliter, A. L., & Sherwood, A. (1993). Race and gender comparisons: I Hemodynamic responses to a series of stressors. *Health Psychology, 12,* 354–365.

Luscher, T. F., & Vanhoutte, P. M. (1990). *The endothelium: Modulator of cardiovascular function.* Boca Raton, FL: CRC Press.

Mahoney, L. T., Schieken, R. M., Clarke, W. R., & Lauer, R. M. (1988). Left ventricular mass and exercise responses predict future blood pressure: The Muscatine Study. *Hypertension, 12,* 206–213.

Malpass, D., Treiber, F. A., Turner, J. R., Davis, H., Thompson, W., Levy, M., & Strong, W. B. (1997). Relationships between children's cardiovascular stress responses and resting cardiovascular functioning one-year later. *International Journal of Psychophysiology, 25,* 139–144.

Manuck, S. B. (1994). Cardiovascular reactivity in cardiovascular disease: "Once more unto the breach." *International Journal of Behavioral Medicine, 1,* 4–31.

Manuck, S. B, Kamarck, T. W., Kasprowicz, A. S., & Waldstein, S. R. (1993). Stability and patterning of behaviorally evoked cardiovascular reactivity. In J. Blascovich & E. S. Katkin (Eds.), *Cardiovascular reactivity to psychological stress and disease* (pp. 111–134). Washington, DC: APA.

Manuck, S. B., Kasprowicz, A. L., & Muldoon, M. F. (1990). Behaviorally evoked cardiovascular reactivity and hypertension: Conceptual issues and potential associations. *Annals of Behavioral Medicine, 12,* 17–29.

Manuck, S. B., Morrison, R. L., Bellack, A. S., & Polefrone, J. M. (1985). Behavioral factors in hypertension: Cardiovascular responsivity, anger and social competence. In M. Chesney & R. Rosenman (Eds.), *Anger and hostility in cardiovascular and behavior disorders* (pp. 149–172). Washington, DC: Hemisphere Publishing Corporation.

Matthews, A., Davis, M., Stoney, C., Owens, J., & Caggiula, A. (1991). Does the gender relevance of the stressor influence sex differences in psychophysiological responses? *Health Psychology, 10,* 112–120.

Matthews, K., Rakaczky, C., Stoney, C., & Manuck, S. (1987). Are cardiovascular responses to behavioral stressors a stable individual difference variable in childhood? *Psychophysiology, 24,* 464–473.

Matthews, K. A., Gump, B. B., Block, D. R., & Allen, M. T. (1997). Does background stress heighten or dampen children's cardiovascular responses to acute stress? *Psychosomatic Medicine, 59,* 488–496.

Matthews, K. A., Manuck, S. B., & Saab, P. G. (1986). Cardiovascular responses of adolescents during a naturally occurring stressor and their behavioral and psychophysiological predictors. *Psychophysiology, 23,* 198–209.

Matthews, K. A., & Stoney, C. M. (1988). Influences of sex and age on cardiovascular responses during stress. *Psychosomatic Medicine, 50,* 46–56.

Matthews, K. A., Weiss, S. M., Detre, T., Dembroski, T. M., Falkner, B., Manuck, S. B., & Williams, R. B., Jr. (1986). *Handbook of stress, reactivity, and cardiovascular disease.* New York: Wiley.

Matthews, K. A., Woodall, K. A., & Stoney, C. M. (1990). Changes in and stability of cardiovascular responses to behavioral stress: Results from a four-year longitudinal study of children. *Child Development, 61,* 1134–1144.

Matthews, K. A., Woodall, K. L., & Allen, M. T. (1993). Cardiovascular reactivity to stress predicts future blood pressure status. *Hypertension, 22,* 479–485.

McCann, B. S., & Matthews, K. A. (1988). Influences of potential for hostility, Type A behavior, and parental history of hypertension on adolescents' cardiovascular responses during stress. *Psychophysiology, 25,* 503–511.

McGrath, J. J., & O'Brien, W. H. (2001). Pediatric impedance cardiography: Temporal stability and intertask consistency. *Psychophysiology, 38,* 479–484.

Mensah, G. A., Liao, Y., & Cooper, R. S. (1995). Left ventricular hypertrophy as a risk factor in patients with or without coronary artery disease. *Cardiovascular Risk Factors, 5,* 67–74.

Meredith, I. T., Yeung, A. C., & Weidinger, F. F. (1993). Role of impaired endothelium-dependent vasodilation in ischemic manifestations of coronary artery disease. *Circulation, 87,* 56–66.

Murdison, K. A., Treiber, F. A., Mensah, G., Davis, H., Thompson, W., & Strong, W. B. (1998). Prediction of left ventricular mass in youth with family histories of essential hypertension. *American Journal of the Medical Sciences, 315,* 118–123.

Murphy, J. K. (1992). Psychophysiological responses to stress in children and adolescents. In P. M. La Greca, L. J. Siegal, J. L. Wallander, & C. E. Walker (Eds.), *Advances in pediatric psychology: Stress and coping in child health* (pp. 44–71). New York: Guilford.

Murphy, J. K., Alpert, B. S., Moes, D. M., & Somes, G. W. (1986). Race and cardiovascular reactivity: A neglected relationship. *Hypertension, 8,* 1075–1083.

Murphy, J. K., Alpert, B. S., & Walker, S. S. (1992). Ethnicity, pressor reactivity, and children's blood pressure: Five years of observation. *Hypertension, 20,* 327–332.

Murphy, J. K., Alpert, B. S., Walker, S. S., & Willey, E. S. (1991). Children's cardiovascular reactivity: Stability of racial differences and relation to subsequent blood pressure over a one-year period. *Psychophysiology, 28,* 447–457.

Murphy, J. K., Alpert, B. S., Walker, S. S., & Willey, E. S. (1994). Consistency of ethnic differences in children's pressor reactivity 1987 to 1992. *Hypertension, 23,* 152–155.

Murphy, J. K., Alpert, B. S., Willey, E. S., Christman, J. V., Sexton, J. E., & Harshfield, G. A. (1989). Modulation of pressor responses by fitness: Racial differences among children. *American Journal of Hypertension, 2,* 25A.

Murphy, J. K., Alpert, B. S., Willey, E. S., & Somes, G. W. (1988). Cardiovascular reactivity to psychological stress in healthy children. *Psychophysiology, 25,* 144–152.

Murphy, J. K., Stoney, C. M., Alpert, B. S., & Walker, S. S. (1995). Gender and ethnicity in children's cardiovascular reactivity: 7 years of study. *Health Psychology, 14,* 48–55.

Musante, L., Raunikar, R. A., Treiber, F., Davis, H., Dysart, J., Levy, M., & Strong, W. B. (1994). Consistency of children's hemodynamic responses to laboratory stressors. *International Journal of Psychophysiology, 17,* 65–71.

Musante, L., Treiber, F. A., Strong, W. B., & Levy, M. (1990). Family history of hypertension and cardiovascular reactivity to forehead cold stimulation in black male children. *Journal of Psychosomatic Research, 34,* 111–116.

Musante, L., Turner, J. R., Treiber, F. A., Davis, H., & Strong, W. B. (1996). Moderators of ethnic differences in vasoconstrictive reactivity in youth. *Ethnicity and Disease, 6,* 224–234.

National High Blood Pressure Education Program. National High Blood Pressure Education Program Working Group Report on Primary Prevention of Hypertension. (1993). *Archives of Internal Medicine, 153,* 186–208.

National High Blood Pressure Education Program National High Blood Pressure Education Program Working Group on Hypertension Control in Children and Adolescents. (1996). Update on the 1987 task force report on high blood pressure in children and adolescents: A working group report. *Pediatrics, 98,* 649–658.

Newman, J. D., McGarvey, S. T., & Steele, M. S. (1999). Longitudinal association of cardiovascular reactivity and blood pressure in Samoan adolescents. *Psychosomatic Medicine, 61,* 243–249.

Newman, W. P., Freedman, D. S., Voors, A. W., Gard, P. D., Srinivasan, S. R., Cresanta, J. L., Williamson, G. D., Webber, L. S., & Berenson, G. S. (1986). Relation of serum lipoprotein levels and systolic blood pressure to early atherosclerosis: The Bogalusa Heart Study. *New England Journal of Medicine, 314,* 138–144.

Noll, G., Wenzel, R. R., Schneider, M., Oesch, V., Binggeli, C., Shaw, S., Weidmann, P., & Luscher, T. F. (1996). Increased activation of sympathetic nervous system and endothelin by mental stress in normotensive offspring of hypertensive parents. *Circulation, 93,* 866–869.

Nora, J. J., Lortscher, R. H., Spangler, R. D., Nora, A. H., & Kimberling, W. J. (1980). Genetic-epidemiologic study of early onset ischemic heart disease. *Circulation, 61,* 503–508.

Panza, J. A., Casino, P. R., Kilcoyne, C. M., & Quyyumi, A. A. (1993). Role of endothelium-derived nitric oxide in the abnormal endothelium-dependent vascular relaxation of patients with essential hypertension. *Circulation, 87,* 1468–1474.

Papavassiliou, D. P., Treiber, F. A., Strong, W. B., Malpass, M. D., & Davis H. (1996). Anthropometric, demographic and cardiovascular predictors of left ventricular mass in young children. *American Journal of Cardiology, 78,* 323–326.

Parker, F. C., Croft, J. B., Cresanta, J. L., Freedman, D. S., Burke, G. L., Webber, L. S., & Berenson, G. S. (1987). The association between cardiovascular response tasks and future blood pressure levels in children: Bogalusa Heart Study. *Circulation, 113,* 1174–1179.

PDAY Research Group. (1990). Relationships of atherosclerosis in young men to serum lipoprotein cholesterol concentrations and smoking: A preliminary report from the Pathobiological Determinants of Atherosclerosis in Youth (PDAY) Research Group. *Journal of the American Medical Association, 264,* 3018–3024.

Pflieger, K. L., Treiber, F. A., Davis, H., McCaffrey, F. M., Raunikar, R. A., & Strong, W. B. (1994). The effect of adiposity on children's left ventricular mass and geometry and haemodynamic responses to stress. *International Journal of Obesity, 18,* 117–122.

Platt, R. (1967). The influence of heredity. In J. Stamler, R. Stamler, & T. N. Pullman (Eds.), *The epidemiology of hypertension* (pp. 9–15). New York: Grune & Stratton.

Polderman, K. H., Steouwer, C. D. A., van Kamp, G. P., Dekker, G. A., Verheugt, F. W. A., & Gooren, L. J. G. (1993). Influence of sex hormones on plasma endothelin levels. *Annals of Internal Medicine, 118,* 429–432.

Radice, M., Alli, C., Avanzini, F., Di Tullio, M., Mariotti, G., Taioli, E., Zussino, A., & Folli, G. (1986). Left ventricular structure and function in normotensive adolescents with a genetic predisposition of hypertension. *American Heart Journal, 111,* 115–120.

Resnicow, K. (1993). School-based obesity prevention: Population versus high-risk interventions. In C. L. Williams & S. Y. S. Kimm (Eds.), *Prevention and treatment of childhood obesity* (pp. 154–166). Annals of the New York Academy of Sciences.

Riley, W., Freedman, D., Higgs, N., Barnes, R., Zinkgraf, S., & Berenson, G. (1986). Decreased arterial elasticity associated with CV disease risk factors in the young. *Arteriosclerosis, 6,* 378–386.

Roncaglioni, M. C., Santoro, L., D'Avanzo, B., Negri, E., Nobili, A., Ahedda, A., Pietropaolo, F., Franzosi, M. G., LaVecchia, C., & Feruglio, G. A. (1992). Role of family history in patients with myocardial infarction: An Italian case-control study. *Circulation, 85,* 2065–2072.

Ross, R. (1993). The pathogenesis of atherosclerosis: A perspective for the 1990s. *Nature, 362,* 801–809.

Saab, P. G., Llabre, M. M., Hurwitz, B. E., Frame, C. A., Reineke, K. J., Fins, A. I., McCalla, J., Cieply, L. K., & Schneiderman, N. (1992). Myocardial and peripheral vascular responses to behavioral challenges and their stability in Black and White Americans. *Psychophysiology, 29,* 384–397.

Sallis, J. F., Dimsdale, J. E., & Caine, C. (1988). Blood pressure reactivity in children. *Journal of Psychosomatic Research, 32,* 1–12.

Schieken, R. M., Clarke, W. R., & Lauer, R. M. (1981). Left ventricular hypertrophy in children with blood pressures in the upper quintile of the distribution: The Muscatine Study. *Hypertension, 3,* 669–675.

Schneiderman, N. (1987). Psychophysiologic factors in atherogenesis and coronary artery disease. *Circulation, 76,* 41–47.

Schneiderman, N., & Skyler, J. S. (1996). Insulin metabolism, sympathetic nervous system regulation, and coronary heart disease prevention. In K. Orth-Gomer & N. Schneiderman (Eds.), *Behavioral medicine approaches to cardiovascular disease prevention* (pp. 105–133). Mahwah, NJ: Lawrence Erlbaum Associates.

Schneiderman, N., Weiss, S. M., & Kaufman, P. G. (1989). *Handbook of research methods in cardiovascular behavioral medicine.* New York: Plenum.

Sherwood, A., & Turner, J. R. (1995). Hemodynamic responses during psychological stress: Implications for studying disease processes. *International Journal of Behavioral Medicine, 2,* 193–218.

Sorensen, K. E., Celermajer, D. S., Georgakopoulos, D., Hatcher, G., Betteridge, J., & Deanfield, J. E. (1994). Impairment of endothelium-dependent dilation is an early event in children with familial hypercholesterolemia, and is related to the Lp(a) level. *Journal of Clinical Investigation, 93,* 50–55.

Stamler, R., Stamler, J., Riedlinger, W. F., Algera, G., & Roberts, R. H. (1979). Family (parental) history and prevalence of hypertension: Results of a nationwide screening program. *Journal of the American Medical Association, 241,* 43–46.

Stary, H. S. (1989). Evolution and progression of atherosclerotic lesions in coronary arteries of children and young adults. *Arteriosclerosis, 9,* 19–32.

Stoney, C. M., Davis, M. C., & Matthews, K. A. (1987). Sex differences in physiological responses to stress and in coronary heart disease: A causal link? *Psychophysiology, 24,* 127–131.

Strong, W. B., Deckelbaum, R. J., Gidding, S. S., Kavey, R. E., Washington, R., Wilmore, J. H., & Perry, C. L. (1992). Integrated cardiovascular health promotion in childhood. *Circulation, 85,* 1638–1650.

Strong, W. B., & Kelder, S. H. (1996). Pediatric preventive cardiology. In J. E. Manson, P. M. Ridker, J. M. Gaziano, & G. H. Hennekens (Eds.), *Prevention of myocardial infarction* (pp. 433–459). New York: Oxford University Press.

Strong, W. B., Miller, M. D., Striplin, M., & Salehbhai, M. (1978). Blood pressure response to isometric and dynamic exercise in healthy black children. *American Journal of Diseases of Children, 132,* 587–591.

Taddei, S., Virdis, A., Mattei, P., Ghiadoni, L., Sudano, I., & Salvetti, A. (1996). Defective L-Arginine-Nitric Oxide pathway in offspring of essential hypertensive patients. *Circulation, 94,* 1298–1303.

Taras, H. L., & Sallis, J. F. (1992). Blood pressure reactivity in young children: Comparing three stressors. *Developmental and Behavioral Pediatrics, 13,* 41–45.

Thompson, W. O., Treiber, F. A., Johnson, M. H., & Davis, H. (1997). Temporal stability of ambulatory blood pressure (ABP) in youth with family history of hypertension. *Annals of Behavioral Medicine, 19,* 168.

Treiber, F., Davis, H., Thompson, W., Levy, M., & Strong, W. (1997). Blood pressure (BP) responsivity to stress predict resting BP four years later in youth. *Annals of Behavioral Medicine, 19,* 169.

Treiber, F., Del Rosario, J., Davis, H., Gutin, B., & Strong, W. B. (1997). *Cardiovascular stress responses predict cardiovascular functioning: A four-year follow-up.* Children and Exercise XIX (pp. 366–372). London: Chapman-Hall.

Treiber, F. A., Jackson, R. W., Davis, H., Pollock, J. S., Kapuku, G., Mensah, G. A., & Pollock, D. M. (2000). Racial differences in Endothelin-1 at rest and in response to acute stress in adolescent males. *Hypertension, 35,* 722–725.

Treiber, F. A., McCaffrey, F., Musante, L., Rhodes, T., Davis, H., Strong, W. B., & Levy, M. (1993). Ethnicity, family history of hypertension and patterns of hemodynamic reactivity in boys. *Psychosomatic Medicine, 55,* 70–77.

Treiber, F. A., McCaffrey, F., Pflieger, K., Raunikar, R. A., Strong, W. B., & Davis, H. (1993). Determinants of left ventricular mass in normotensive children. *American Journal of Hypertension, 6,* 505–513.

Treiber, F. A., McCaffrey, F., Strong, W. B., Davis, H., & Baranowski, T. (1991). Automated exercise blood pressure measurements in children: A preliminary study. *Pediatric Exercise Science, 3,* 290–299.

Treiber, F. A., Murphy, J. K., Davis, H., Raunikar, A., Pflieger, K., & Strong, W. B. (1994). Pressor reactivity, ethnicity, and 24-hour ambulatory monitoring in children from hypertensive families. *Behavioral Medicine, 20,* 133–142.

Treiber, F. A., Musante, L., Braden, D. S., Arensman, F., Strong, W. B., Levy, M., & Leverett, S. (1990). Racial differences in hemodynamic responses to the cold face stimulus in children and adults. *Psychosomatic Medicine, 5,* 286–296.

Treiber, F. A., Musante, L., Kapuku, G., Davis, C., Litaker, M., & Davis, H. (2001). Cardiovascular (CV) responsivity and recovery to acute stress and future CV functioning in youth with family histories of CV disease: A 4-year longitudinal study. *International Journal of Psychophysiology, 41,* 65–74.

Treiber, F. A., Raunikar, R. A., Davis, H., Fernandez, T., Levy, M., & Strong, W. B. (1994). One year stability and prediction of cardiovascular functioning at rest and during laboratory stressors in youth with family histories of hypertension. *International Journal of Behavioral Medicine, 1,* 335–353.

Treiber, F. A., Strong, W. B., Arensman, F. W., Forrest, T., Davis, H., & Musante, L. (1991). Family history of myocardial infarction and hemodynamic responses to exercise in young black boys. *American Journal of Diseases of Children, 145,* 1029–1033.

Treiber, F. A., Turner, J. R., Davis, H., Thompson, W., Levy, M., & Strong, W. B. (1996). Young children's cardiovascular stress responses predict resting cardiovascular functioning 2 1/2 years later. *Journal of Cardiovascular Risk, 3,* 95–100.

Turner, J. R. (1994). *Cardiovascular reactivity and stress: Patterns of physiological response.* New York: Plenum.

Turner, J. R., Sherwood, A., & Light, K. C. (1994). Intertask consistency of hemodynamic responses to laboratory stressors in a biracial sample of men and women. *International Journal of Psychophysiology, 17,* 159–164.

Urbina, E. M., Gidding, S. S., Bao, W., Pickoff, A. S., Berdusis, K., & Berenson, G. S. (1995). Effect of body size, ponderosity, and blood pressure on left ventricular growth in children and young adults in the Bogalusa Heart Study. *Circulation, 91,* 2400–2406.

Van Doornen, L. J. P., & De Geus, E. J. C. (1989). Aerobic fitness and the cardiovascular response to stress. *Psychophysiology, 26,* 17–28.

Verhaaren, H. A., Shieken, R. M., Mosteller, M., Hewitt, J. K., Eaves, L. J., & Nance, W. E. (1991). Bivariate genetic analysis of left ventricular mass and weight in pubertal twins (The Medical College of Virginia Twin Study). *American Journal of Cardiology, 68,* 661–668.

Visser, M. C., Grobbee, D. E., & Hofman, A. (1987). Determinants of rise in blood pressure in normotensive children. *Journal of Hypertension, 5,* 367–370.

Weber, K. T., Sun, Y., & Guarda, E. (1994). Structural remodeling in hypertensive heart disease and the role of hormones. *Hypertension, 23,* 869–877.

Whelton, P. K., He, J., & Appel, L. J. (1996). Treatment and prevention of hypertension. In J. E. Manson, P. M. Ridker, J. M. Gaziano, & C. H. Hennekens (Eds.), *Prevention of myocardial infarction* (pp. 154–171). New York: Oxford.

Wolinsky, H., Goldfischer, S., Daly, M. M., Kasak, L. E., & Coltoff-Schiller, B. (1975). Arterial lysomes and connective tissue in primate atherosclerosis and hypertension. *Circulatory Research, 36,* 553–561.

Wood, D. L., Sheps, S. G., Elveback, L. R., & Schirger, A. (1984). Cold pressor test as a predictor of hypertension. *Hypertension, 6,* 301–306.

Woodall, K. L., & Matthews, K. A. (1989). Familial environment associated with Type A behaviors and psychophysiological responses to stress in children. *Health Psychology, 8,* 403–426.

Wright, L. B., Treiber, F. A., Davis, H., & Strong, W. B. (1996). Relationship of John Henryism to cardiovascular functioning at rest and during stress in youth. *Annals of Behavioral Medicine, 18,* 146–150.

Wright, L. B., Treiber, F. A., Davis, H., Strong, W. B., Levy, M., Van Huss, E., & Batchelor, C. (1993). Relationship between family environment and children's hemodynamic responses to stress: A longitudinal evaluation. *Behavioral Medicine, 19,* 115–121.

Wright, L. B., Treiber, F. A., Davis, H. C., & Strong, W. B. (1997). Psychosocial and lifestyle predictors of cardiovascular reactivity in youth with family history of hypertension. In N. Armstrong, B. Kirby, & J. Welsman (Eds.), *Children and exercise* (pp. 390–397). London: E & FN Spon.

Zahka, K. G., Neill, C. A., Kidd, L., Cutilletta, M. A., & Cutilletta, A. F. (1981). Cardiac involvement in adolescent hypertension: Echocardiographic determination of myocardial hypertrophy. *Hypertension, 3,* 664–668.

Zeiher, A., Drexler, H., Wollschlager, H., & Just, H. (1991). Modulation of coronary vasomotor tone in humans. *Circulation, 83,* 391–401.

PART II

Related Issues

CHAPTER 6

Family Considerations

Margaret P. Shepard and Margaret M. Mahon

C aring for a child with a chronic condition also involves caring for the child's family. The family has been consistently recognized in the context of care, often performing many complex medical procedures in addition to facilitating the child's social, emotional and developmental needs. The role of the family as members of the health care team and as essential participants in critical decision making processes is less well established. In this chapter, some of the ways families grow in relation to, and are challenged by, their experiences with a child with a chronic condition are examined. In addition, specific recommendations for clinicians are made to optimize family success in their experiences of caring for children with chronic conditions.

The definition of family and the expectations of family members vary from culture to culture. Any definition of the family should include the following concepts: generational and permanent relationships, a nurturing and caregiving orientation, emotional intensity, a mixture of qualitative and quantitative purposes, altruistic values, and a nurturing form of governance (Beutler, Burr, Bahr, & Herrin, 1989). The family is the environment within which the child's needs for growth and development can be met. A well-functioning family is one in which the members continue to grow and develop (Shepard, 1992). Moreover, the family influences individual members' expressions of illness and health through the processes of socialization and the transmission of basic values, beliefs, attitudes, hopes, and aspirations.

The family is a unique group that can be represented by many different configurations of its members. Variation in family structure does not necessarily mean weaker families, although variations do require the clinician to have a greater awareness and sensitivity to differences within individual families and within society. Relationships within the family, rather than structure or type of family, are much greater predictors of outcomes for children (Visher & Visher, 1995). Each family is defined by individual, ethnic, and cultural influences. The clinician should identify the roles each family member fulfills, as well as the family's perception of their strengths and weaknesses.

FAMILY CRISIS AND ADAPTATION

A chronic condition is one that is not only long term but is either not curable or has residual features that result in limitation(s) requiring special assistance or adaptation in function (Eiser, 1993; Hayes, 1997; Jessop & Stein, 1985). The condition need not be permanent, serious, or obvious. On the other hand, some chronic conditions are irreversible, serious, and require comprehensive care. Some are fatal. A child with a chronic condition may be seriously impaired from birth, may have a transitory condition from which recovery is complete, or may have any degree of severity in between. Furthermore, a diagnosis is not always indicative of the severity of a child's condition. For example, asthma, the most common chronic condition of childhood, may severely affect a child's ability to function on a daily basis or may cause only occasional short-term disability.

Many families perceive the early diagnostic period and acute exacerbations of the child's illness as times of crisis. All crises challenge family coping; the family must learn to adapt. The way the family perceives the situation, problem-solving strategies, coping repertoire, and usual patterns of functioning will moderate the family's ability to adapt to the new situation (McCubbin, 1993). The attempt to adapt leaves the family stronger, weaker, or dissolved. Clinical assessment of the family's response to the chronic condition should include an evaluation of the situation in the context of other family changes and stresses. For example, the family whose newborn has a condition necessitating surgery or other treatment is dealing with the birth of a newborn and the newborn's chronic condition.

One family member's personal situation has an effect on all other family members. A chronic condition in a child not only affects that child but has ramifications for all members of the family system (Kazak, 1989a). Having a child with a chronic condition is stressful; however, families who have a child with a chronic condition do not suffer a noticeable excess of dysfunction relative to other families (Cadman et al., 1991; Hostler, 1991). Families are not only managing the specific event that brings them to the attention of the health care system, but they are also managing other stresses from all areas of work and family life. An excess accumulation of family demands will adversely affect family adaptation (McCubbin, 1993; Patterson & McCubbin, 1983).

Any family's functional level will not be static; rather, the functional level may fluctuate over time. These changes in functional ability relate to the myriad stresses that impinge on the system, as well as the family's ability to cope (Gallo & Knafl, 1998; McCubbin, 1993). Interventions with families, then, can only be made with family input regarding stressors, not only related to caring for a child with a chronic condition, but also how these interact with concurrent albeit unrelated stressors.

FAMILY RESPONSES TO THE DIAGNOSIS OF A CHRONIC CONDITION

The diagnosis of a chronic condition is a stressful time, often causing disequilibrium within families. Parents have described the time between their initial awareness of the child's symptoms and the leveling of a diagnosis as overwhelming, characterized by uncertainty and a sense of "groping in the dark" (Horner, 1997). The family response may include shock, disbelief, denial (Holaday, 1984; Parker, 1996), disgust, relief, guilt, despair, hate, rage, or confusion (Hobbs, Perrin, & Ireys, 1985). Parents are likely to grieve the healthy child they envisioned (Solnit & Stark, 1962; Meyers & Weitzman, 1991).

Parents may experience great relief when the diagnosis is made as it relieves some of the uncertainty. Some parents, however, describe new areas of uncertainty. Parents may wonder how the condition will effect the family as a whole and each of the individual members. Some may find that their taken-for-granted world has been destroyed, as they begin to lean to manage under very uncertain conditions (Cohen, 1993). Some factors that affect the responses of parents and others are (1) the visibility of the condition, (2) whether there are functional limitations or not (Silver, Westbrook, & Stein, 1998), (3) the presence or absence of mental retardation, (4) the expectation of pain for the child, (5) the uncertainty about changes in the condition, (6) the parents' experience with others who have chronic conditions, and (7) the preconceived ideas about the condition that might engender reactions that are incongruent with the reality of the condition.

The family's perception of the impact of the illness on the family system will affect the level of family functioning and subsequent responses to the diagnosis of a chronic condition. Family structure, previous experiences managing stressful events, requirements of the child's condition, and other factors unique to each family will also influence the family's experience.

To intervene optimally, the clinician should consider not only the facts, requirements, and nuances of each condition, but the resources and coping patterns of each family. To assess family coping the clinician should inquire about the family's previous experiences with stressful events and how they were managed. Concurrent stresses in the family and what resources are available to meet the perceived demands also need to be explored. Resources may include financial and material goods as well as a support network of family and friends. Families managing a great deal of stresses with limited resources may experience greater challenge than families with fewer stresses or more resources.

Another resource to facilitate family coping is accurate information about the condition, treatment options, and community resources such as adaptive equipment and support services. The diagnosis sets some parents on a search for information about the condition, including causes, treatments, and effects. This quest for information is usually very appropriate and should be supported as part of the family's efforts to cope. Parents are obtaining knowledge about the condition, which is the first step in having some control over the situation (Hobbs, Perrin, & Ireys, 1985; Swallow & Jacoby, 2001). It may be helpful to accompany the family on a predischarge home visit to help prepare for the child's needs (Bakewell-Sachs et al., 2000.) A thorough assessment of the home environment can facilitate parent teaching and may help identify unanticipated situations. Use of the internet has greatly increased the range of information to which families have access. As a result, clinicians may be required to clarify information and respond to sophisticated questions posed by family members. Clinicians should periodically update their knowledge of information sources available on the internet so they can direct families to appropriate resources and to warn them about inflammatory or inaccurate internet sites.

Ultimately, many families will also search for some level of meaning by asking the question "why me?" Often they will identify religious, philosophic, or scientific reasons for the child's condition (Holaday, 1984). Family functioning can be enhanced if parents have a more positive than negative interpretation, and are able to define the chronic condition and resultant situations within a previously existing personal, medical-scientific and/or religious world view (Coyne, 1997; Venters, 1981). Parents should be encouraged to discuss their search for meaning with one another as well as with the clinician, other families in the same situation, or with a supportive friend.

While far less uncommon, and no longer a new disease, the diagnosis of HIV in a newborn has some unique implications. Often, the diagnosis of HIV in a newborn becomes associated with the new diagnosis of other family members. Parents' reactions include not only the overwhelming response to the child's life threatening illness, but also the awareness that the parent might die before the child, leaving the child orphaned. Care concerns may be further complicated by parental guilt, continued addiction and/or other compromised lifestyle behaviors. Parents of children with HIV, whether HIV (–) or HIV (+) are likely to have clinical significant stress. Parents who are HIV+ are more likely to perceive themselves has having poorer health, with fewer social supports, and are likely to be *less* pessimistic about the future of the child and the family (Amodei, Madrigal, Catala, Aranda-Naranjo, & German, 1997). All of this occurs in addition to the family's reaction to having a baby—in itself a very stressful situation.

Appropriately, the prognosis of the condition affects the response. If a condition is, or might be life threatening, a terror about the child's possible or impending death is likely to pervade the initial reactions. Although it is the pattern of many health care providers *not* to discuss death while there is possibility of a cure, this is not helpful for two reasons. First, fear of a child's death is likely to be in the forefront of the parents' thinking. Other things planned or taught will be heard only through this veil of fear. It is only after dealing with this fear that other planning and interventions can be most effective. Second, acknowledging the possibility of death, using the word, shows families that the clinician is willing to discuss the subject. One might say, "Yes, the long-term outcome is not good. But the treatments we have are very good, and your child can have a very good quality of life for several years. When it comes time to focus more on the death, I will tell you. Now we have to focus on what we can treat, and how it will be done." This honesty provides a strong foundation for an open relationship with the family.

Role of the Clinician

When a chronic condition is diagnosed, the focus of the family often narrows and becomes very disease focused. Whether caring for a newborn or an older child, the clinician should consider several important guidelines. First, family-centered care and a trusting relationship with the clinician are pivotal to successful treatment (American Academy of Pediatrics [AAP], 2001; Cohen & Wambolt, 2000). Family-centered care includes a respectful and accepting emotional climate developed between family and clinicians. Parents are less likely to respond positively when the clinician uses a critical tone or makes critical comments.

Sometimes family-centered care can lead to an ethical dilemma. For example, parents may elect to pursue unconventional treatments or to forgo recommended interventions. In these situations clinicians must be aware of their personal value and professional guidelines so that there can be effective negotiations with families. The clinician must balance respect for the parents' choices with knowledge of the best medical options. Complementary and Alternative Medicines (CAM) have been increasingly integrated into mainstream treatment options (AAP, 2001). In fact, many CAMs have proven efficacious. Many CAMs, however, have not been rigorously tested. Furthermore, choices made by parents that are known to be harmful to the child—for example, attempting dietary modifications in lieu of insulin therapy for a child with Type 1 diabetes, may necessitate the clinician taking more aggressive action.

Second, provide families with accurate, current, concrete information. Families should be given as much information as is immediately needed, but not much more. Parents should receive information in sufficient time to be full and active participants in the decision-making process. An insufficient understanding of the child's illness and treatment needs has been linked to poor adherence and excess risk for acute exacerbations of the condition (Dosa, Boeing, & Kanter, 2001). Encourage families to ask questions and then take the time to answer them. Provide information in writing or allow them to tape record information sessions. One must also consider that in certain cultures it is considered inappropriate to ask questions of health care providers. Children should be given developmentally appropriate information. Gauge the level of information to meet the child's and family's needs, and periodically assess how each is responding to and using the information. Information and written material that is overly simplistic, too complex or inappropriately timed is not helpful and may ultimately alienate the family.

Third, help the family put the diagnosis in perspective. This may be challenging, but can be very helpful for families. Do not make assumptions about how the family is responding to their new situation. Ascertain what expectations and knowledge the family already has. If there are misconceptions, clarify them. In addition, identify the child's strengths. For example, complement the cheerful temperament of the child with trisomy 21. Do not attempt to minimize the seriousness of the situation; rather focus on the child as an individual with many of the same needs and strengths as other children.

There are no right or wrong responses for family members at the time of diagnosis. The coping strategies of families are rich and diverse. They may reflect ethnic or other cultural values unfamiliar to the clinician. Different cultural and religious belief systems should be explored, understood and accepted by the clinician (Hostler, 1991). The clinician should look for cues from the family concerning their readiness to learn, their obstacles to accepting the diagnosis, and their unique fears or stresses and respond to these cues in a supportive manner. Family strengths and prior coping patterns must be considered when intervening with families. Because ultimate care for the child resides with the family, the family must be a part of, and not merely the subject or recipient of interventions. This means using and respecting the knowledge the family has acquired, not only about the condition, but also about the child and how that child is likely to respond. Empowerment of the family by providers can enhance the quality of life of the family (Hartley & Fuller, 1997).

Family Roles and Responsibilities

The management of a chronic condition is a family affair, however, it rarely falls equally on family caregivers. It is now well documented that the mother is usually identified as the one primarily responsible for the day-to-day care and management of the child (Gallo & Knafl, 1998; Glazer, 1990; Jessop, Reissman, & Stein, 1988; Kazak, 1989a). Some mothers give up employment to care for their child, due as much to the demands of medical treatment as to the stresses of parenting a child with a chronic condition (Mastroyannopoulou, Stallard, Lewis, & Lenton, 1997; Stein et al., 1989). Because of limited day care for children with chronic conditions, some mothers who might otherwise be employed are forced to stay at home (Rearson, Urban, Baker, McBride, Tuttle, & Jawad, 2000). Although there can be numerous stressors, many mothers evaluate their caregiving experience as very positive.

Negative psychological sequelae for parents have been the focus of numerous studies over the years. Recently, researchers have identified a fairly consistent relationship between caring for a child with a chronic condition and increased *parenting stress*. Silver, Westbrook, and Stein (1998) found that when the chronic condition included functional limitations, the parents experienced greater distress. Based on a review of the literature, Ievers and Drotar (1996) concluded that parents of children with cystic fibrosis experienced greater stress and burden, yet parenting behaviors and family functioning were similar to those in healthy control groups. Frank and colleagues (1998) compared 114 families of children with diabetes with 88 families with healthy children. Their results supported a relationship between the chronic condition, mothers' depression, parenting distress for both mothers and fathers, and a passive style of family coping. Interestingly, in this study, the children's emotional and behavioral functioning were not related to their chronic condition; rather, the children's adjustment was associated with maternal depression and parenting distress. Similarly, Frankel and Wambolt (1998) found that parental emotional distress was associated with greater impact of the illness on the family system in a study of 70 families with children with asthma. Jessop, Reissman, and Stein (1988) found a relationship between functional status of the child and the mother's symptoms of distress; however, these authors concluded that maternal symptoms may have a stronger relationship to the stresses experienced than to the child's actual functional level.

It would certainly be inaccurate to deny that caring for a child with a chronic condition is associated with unique stressors and hardships. Nonetheless, more recently, researchers' have uncovered fewer negative sequelae than were previously supposed. In addition, considerable variations in outcomes (Drotar, 1997; Wallander & Varni, 1998) and an array of protective factors associated with family functioning have been identified. For example, Kell and colleagues (1998) studied 80 adolescents with sickle cell disease and found that higher family competence was associated with better adjustment in the children; these relations were particularly true for younger adolescents and girls. In a study of children with kidney disease, better family adjustment was associated with less parenting stress and fewer behavior problems (Shepard, 1992; Soliday, Kool, & Lande, 2000). These studies have important implications for the development of interventions for families in which stresses are associated with complex roles and responsibilities.

The parenting stress associated with the chronic condition and/or resultant treatments may bring about behavioral changes that affect the parent's relationship with the child (Sheeran, Marvin, & Pianta, 1997). Age and gender of the child may also affect how mothers perceive the burden of caring for the child. Compared with mothers of daughters, mothers of sons with sickle cell disease were usually more involved in caregiving, more likely to intervene to protect their child's health, and expressed more anxiety over their child's health. Mothers of sons were also more likely to describe their child's health as fragile, and they were more likely to supervise closely and restrict their son's activities (Hill & Zimmerman, 1995). Parents of younger children had more future oriented concerns related to prognosis (Soliday et al., 2000) and care needs, ability to marry and have children (Shepard, 1992).

Families perceive the chronic condition, its effects, and its implications in a variety of ways. Some families are able to integrate the condition as just another part of the daily routine, whereas others perceive it as a feared and loathsome intrusion into their lives. Knafl and colleagues (1993) categorized families' views of chronic illness as a "manageable condition," an "ominous situation," a "hateful restriction," or that the family had a "limited understanding of the condition." These authors explored the interactions of parents' views of their children and parenting philosophies. Parents generally shared similar perceptions of the care demands (Knafl & Zoeller, 2000). There was an interactive effect between the views of those involved in parenting and caregiving. Each family may define the roles and responsibilities of caring for a child with a chronic condition in different, yet equally effective ways. Moreover, as in all families, how the family assigns the roles and responsibilities is likely to change over time due to the changing developmental and environmental demands on the family.

Family Management Styles

Family management style has been conceptualized as the configuration formed by individual family member's definitions of the situation, the management behaviors in which each engages with respect to the chronic illness, and the sociocultural context in which these definitions and behaviors occur (Deatrick, Knafl, & Murphy-Moore, 1999; Knafl, Breitmayer, Gallo, & Zoeller, 1996). Definition of the situation is the subjective meaning of the situation for each person. Management behaviors are the discrete behavioral accommodations that family members use to manage the illness on a daily basis. Recent research by Knafl and colleagues (1996) has identified five distinct family management styles: thriving, accommodating, enduring, struggling, and floundering.

Thriving and accommodative families view the illness situation and the child as "normal." Parents have an accommodative philosophy, confidence in, and a proactive stance toward their ability to manage the illness. Children view themselves as "healthy." Like thriving families, accommodative families view their situation as essentially normal though more negatively than their thriving peers. Accommodative parents may take a more compliant approach to the illness management and may identify more negative consequences related to managing the illness. Enduring families tend to perceive more difficulty and greater negative consequences in their situation. Although the child may be viewed as normal, some families describe their child with a chronic condition as a "tragic figure" thus, parents tend to be more protective of the child. Struggling families are characterized by conflict over how best to manage their child's illness. Struggling parents perceive less support and mutuality from one another; particularly mothers felt they received insufficient support from their spouses. Children in struggling families perceived the illness as a greater intrusion in their lives and as an ongoing source of worry. Floundering families are distinguished by a sense of confusion. Parents define themselves and their situation as negative. They are uncertain about best management approaches. Illness management is perceived as difficult and as a burden. The child is viewed as a tragic figure, however, some children may minimize the impact of the illness on their lives.

It is interesting to consider whether these management styles could be used to describe any parenting situation. That is, the chronic condition is superimposed on a family with its preexisting management style. As such, most parents will continue to parent as they have parented, and most families will function in the style that they have functioned. The research by Knafl and colleagues (1996) was based on families' descriptions of their management style, indicating that the clinician's assessment of family perceptions is valid as at least a baseline assessment. The authors also found, however, that 52% of the participating families described using a different management style at two interviews 1 year apart. Ongoing assessments of the family management style will contribute to targeted interventions based on information about whether challenges to adaptation are due to problems in the family definition of the situation, management approaches, or differences between the parents.

Normalization is the overriding theme that characterizes the successful management process used by many families of children with chronic conditions. Normalization acknowledging the condition and its potential to threaten lifestyle, adapting a "normalcy lens" for defining child and family, engaging in parenting behaviors and family routines that are consistent with the normalcy lens, developing a treatment regimen that is consistent with a normalcy lens, and interacting with others based on a view of the child and the family as normal (Deatrick, Knafl, & Murphy-Moore, 1999). Normalization is an ongoing process of actively accommodating the child's evolving physical, emotional, and social needs (Deatrick, Knafl, & Walsh, 1988). The child is integrated into the mainstream to the greatest extent possible (Holaday, 1984). Acknowledging the condition is essential as the foundation of normalization. There is no denial involved, rather the family is making a statement that "this child is a part of our family, and our family is just like every other family." The child's age and the condition's severity affect the ability of the family to use the process of normalization (Knafl & Deatrick, 1986; Rehm & Franck, 2000).

Normalization is important because it focuses on the child, not on the condition. Most parents who have used normalization techniques have discovered these techniques on their own. Parents may go through a series of stages as they learn to care for their child on a day-to-day basis. In this process family tasks and activities may be reorganized so the illness regime becomes a routine part of family life (Jerret, 1994). The process, however, involves some concrete steps that can be taught. The clinician can demonstrate some of these steps by recognizing the normalcy, the strengths, and the weaknesses of the family system, by being open and supportive concerning the child's condition and treatment, and by actively involving the family in all aspects of care. Reinforcing the family's successful use of these tactics can improve self-esteem and motivate further development.

As the clinician works with families to accommodate the illness and their selected lifestyle, it is helpful to recall that families have successfully demonstrated a variety of approaches to chronic childhood illness management. Gallo and Knafl (1998) identified three predominant approaches: (1) strict adherence, (2) flexible adherence, and (3) selective adherence. Families that follow a strict approach to adherence work closely with health professionals and comply strictly to the prescribed treatment plan. The primary goal in this approach is to control the illness and related symptoms. Families that follow a selective approach to adherence share the goal of illness and symptom control; however, they may develop alternative treatment plans and work independently of professionals. Families that take a flexible approach to adherence focus on a goal of streamlining treatment and making life more livable while maintaining illness control. Flexible parents work closely with health professionals to achieve their goal, however, they are likely to modify treatment plans to achieve their goals.

When the family management approach veers from the prescribed treatment plan, health care providers tend to view these families as noncompliant without considering that the underlying goals for the family and the health care provider may be the same. Awareness of different approaches to managing a child's condition can provide important information about how health care professionals and parents interact as they mutually strive to meet the goals of illness management (Gallo & Knafl, 1998). It may be helpful to encourage families to articulate their goals and family management approaches. This may provide key information by which to intervene more thoughtfully with families based on their approach to treatment as they manage their child's condition on a daily basis.

Siblings

The impact of the chronic condition on siblings can be analyzed in much the same way as other childhood stressors. Many children do not perceive having a sibling with a chronic condition as a significant stressor. Children with a sibling with a chronic condition have been found not to experience greater problems in behavior and social competence (Gallo, Breitmayer, Knafl, & Zoeller, 1992). For some children, having a sibling with a chronic condition engenders feelings of isolation, rejection, anxiety, helplessness, resentment, guilt, or depression. These feelings may be greater at the time of diagnosis, hospitalization, or acute exacerbations of the chronic condition. Siblings often lack information and have decreased access to other family members. Children may perceive an imbalance between the importance of their needs and those of the affected siblings.

There are times when the child with the chronic condition needs increased attention, such as hospitalization. This is often difficult for siblings in several ways. Much has been written about the resentment and inconvenience of such stressors for siblings. It is very important, however, that clinicians recognize that problems in the relationship may have predated the diagnosis. Barbarian and colleagues (1995) found that parents reported 12% of siblings of children with cancer had behavior or affective symptoms before the diagnosis. This increased to 26% after the diagnosis. During hospitalization, 77% of siblings of children with chronic conditions reported feeling stress. In the same sample, 77% of siblings reported feelings of sadness during the hospitalization (Morrison, 1997).

Siblings are directly and immediately affected by the diagnosis of a chronic condition but often lack the ability to control or affect the many and perhaps serious changes within the family. Children often guess about the chronic condition and the resulting health status. They may hear things from friends who received information from their parents. Increasingly, adolescents and even younger siblings access information on the internet. What they overhear or piece together is often much worse than the reality. If the parents are unable to talk to the siblings, it is important that someone else speak with the siblings in a developmentally appropriate way.

The effects of a condition or its treatment, such as hair loss, flatulence, or copious secretions, may be embarrassing for siblings of school age and older. At the same time, children also want to protect the affected sibling from the derisive statements or stares of others. Any feelings of shame and embarrassment are usually not severe, though they can engender simultaneous or subsequent feelings of guilt (Bluebond-Langer, 1996).

Some siblings complain that the child with the chronic condition is treated more leniently. Parents may be unaware that they are treating their children with different standards, or feel that, "Of course I'm not as strict with him. Look at all he has to put up with." This question of discipline is crucial. Quittner and Opipari (1994) concluded that there were both qualitative and quantitative differences in parenting when a child with cystic fibrosis (CF) was in the family, despite the parents' lack of awareness. All children need limits and structure. Discipline supplies both and should be consistent within families and between siblings. It is appropriate for the clinician to question families about methods and consistency of discipline.

Siblings are usually very aware of their negative feelings, which may include anger, feelings of being neglected, fears of causality, contagion, or responsibility, and other founded and unfounded feelings. As a result of their negative feelings, they may experience guilt. It is helpful to tell children that their emotions are acceptable, but at the same time to clarify misconceptions. Clinicians in conjunction with the parents can confirm a sibling's perception that he or she has been receiving less attention and tell the child that it is okay to feel angry about receiving less attention.

Siblings have also described many positive effects from having a sibling with a chronic condition. These include greater maturity, supportiveness and independence (Barbarian et al., 1995). Siblings of children with myelomeningocele were found to have a high degree of empathy and concern for the affected child (Kiburz, 1994). Siblings of children with chronic conditions have been reported to be cooperative and cognitively able to master situations earlier than their peers. Positive responses were even more likely to occur among adolescents and firstborn siblings, and when the sibling's prognosis was less positive (Barbarian et al., 1995).

Among siblings of hospitalized children, children older than 7 years and those with more than one visit to the hospital had more behavioral changes (Morrison, 1997). Older sisters might be called on more often than younger sisters to perform care-giving tasks. Williams, Lorenzo, and Borja (1993) found that siblings of children with chronic conditions had significantly more responsibilities at home, involving both housework and child care. Siblings' perceptions of the home environment are likely to differ from the impressions of their parents (Feeman & Hagen, 1990). This is another reminder that providers should speak directly with siblings, rather than relying on impressions of parents. Siblings' abilities to contribute to family life should be recognized (Kiburz, 1994). Siblings may benefit from being involved in caregiving responsibilities if the sibling is interested in doing so and if the tasks are within their developmental ranges.

Throughout the course of the chronic condition, information for the siblings needs to be updated for two primary reasons. First, what is known about the condition changes, both as the affected child and parents learn more about the condition and because the manifestations of the condition in this particular child might change. Second, the developmental levels of the siblings change, thereby changing their ability to integrate information.

Social Support

A primary need of most families is emotional support and practical help. The amount and type of social support received by families is an essential factor in the family adjustment to the chronic condition (Frankel & Wamboldt, 1998). In general, families receive adequate support from a variety of sources including other family members, friends, and health care providers (Garwick, Patterson, Bennett, & Blum, 1998). Parents, however, may differ on the types of support received from these sources. Both mothers and fathers tend to rely on other family members for emotional and tangible support. Health care providers are perceived as most helpful when informational support is provided (Burke, Handley-Derry, Costello, Kauffmann, & Dillon, 1997; Dokken & Sydnor-Greenberg, 1998). Clinicians should assess the type of support needed before planning supportive interventions.

At the time of diagnosis there is often an influx of concerned people. Tangible types of support that families have found helpful include transportation for siblings, having siblings stay with friends during hospitalizations, providing meals, doing the laundry, running errands, or baby-sitting in the home so that the parents can have some time for personal needs. This latter form of assistance may entail learning care such as cardiopulmonary resuscitation (CPR), use of monitors, or emergency care. It is extremely important that someone in addition to the mother be able and willing to do this. Families usually rely on other family members and close friends to assist them at this time. Offers of support from neighbors and uninformed community members may be perceived as unhelpful. Sometimes, well intended neighbors have made insensitive remarks; suggested that the parents were to blame for their child's condition; and generally lacked adequate knowledge and understanding of the child's condition or treatment (Garwick et al., 1998). Clinicians may help families early in the diagnostic and treatment process by encouraging them to plan for and utilize helpful resources. Parents may benefit from the notion that it is okay to refuse certain types of well intended support from family and friends. Improved social supports benefit the entire family (Hamlett, Pelligrini, & Katz, 1992).

Mothers may perceive and use social supports differently from fathers. For example, mothers may be more critical of, and more dissatisfied with the quality of help received, especially from extended family members and health professionals (Patterson, Garwick, Bennett, & Blum, 1997). Race and ethnicity may also influence the ways families perceive and utilize social supports (Garwick, Kohrman, Wolman, & Blum, 1998). In a comparison study of black families and white families, white families were more likely to identify affective support (e.g., support conveying empathy and understanding) as their primary type of support, whereas black families identified instrumental assistance (e.g., help with other children or transportation) as the primary means of support (Williams, 1993). Clinicians can facilitate family support by identifying the types of support that may be most helpful for the family and by being knowledgeable and culturally sensitive about community resources and parents' groups.

School

The transition to school can be an exciting yet difficult time for families. Regulations such as PL94–142 and 99–457 are important guidance for families in knowing specifics regarding what the child is entitled. Although attendance at school is an indication that the child is like other children and well enough to attend school, many obstacles may need to be overcome in starting and maintaining school participation. While some teachers, administrators, and school systems are eager to be accommodating to children's special needs, others are less willing, and convey their reluctance to families. Furthermore, those who are willing may not perceive themselves as qualified to provide optimal interventions to children with chronic conditions (Mahon, Goldberg, & Washington, 1999b).

Federal regulations stipulate that child with special needs are entitled to an Individualized Education Plan (IEP) and to an education in the least restrictive setting. As advocates for their children, many parents become well informed about the regulations. In today's climate of dwindling public resources, however, school personnel may believe they lack adequate resources to provide effectively for the child's needs. Therefore, families in which a child has a chronic condition are left in a very difficult position. Optimally their child should be in school (AAP Committee on School Health, 2000).

FOSTER CARE

Children with chronic conditions are overrepresented in the foster care system. Children enter foster care for a myriad of reasons, each having to do with a parent's inability or unavailability to provide care. Children enter foster care if a parent has died or is too sick to provide care. Parental illness or disability resulting in foster care includes physical illness, such as HIV, as well as addictions to alcohol or other drugs when that addiction interferes with an ability to provide care. Poverty that results in a lack of food or shelter can also result in foster care. Often these problems interrelate, especially in the areas of addiction, poverty, and HIV. Another major reason for foster care placement is when the child has been abused, either neglected, or physically, emotionally, or sexually abused. Children may be in formal foster care, or may be being raised by extended family.

Foster care exists within the context of complex sociopolitical systems. Many children in foster care have been medically underserved before their placement. Once in foster care, getting the often complex care that they need is very difficult (Blatt & Simms, 1997; Carlson, 1996; Cohen, Nehring, Malm, & Harris, 1995; Rosenfeld at al., 1997). Many of these children have not had adequate primary care, dental care, or mental health care. As a result, they may be deficient in immunizations or an array of undetected conditions. It may also be difficult to obtain an adequate health history due to the transitory lives of many children in foster care.

Foster care parents often have difficulty obtaining services for the children in their care (Barton, 1998). Clinicians can improve access as well as direct health of the child (Blatt & Simms, 1997; Brodie, Berridge, & Beckett, 1997; Carlson, 1996; Cohen et al., 1995). Efforts should focus on three areas: gathering as much data as possible regarding past health and risk factors; compiling a broad and thorough database for the present (recognizing that this is likely to travel with the child); and, being aware of the risk factors of children in foster care, to try to provide for a healthier future.

Long-Term Adaptation

Initial responses of the family system to a chronic condition are often similar to an acute illness. After living with the condition and learning its nuances and management, the family has a more thorough understanding of chronicity. The depth and breadth of understanding may only be shared by the immediate family and a few close friends or extended family members. Relatively simple things such as going out for a meal can become challenging, require additional planning, and may be time limited if a child cannot be away from, for example, suctioning and oxygen for an extended period.

Selected aspects of some chronic conditions are frequently viewed by the parents as disruptive to their relationship with their child (Goldberg & Simmons, 1988). Examples include parents of children with cystic fibrosis who must perform postural drainage, the decreased physical contact that might be required if the child has osteogenesis imperfecta, or the blood testing and insulin injections required by children with diabetes. Parenting a child with a chronic condition involves qualitatively different work than parenting a child without a chronic condition (Deatrick, Knafl, & Walsh, 1988). There is often the assumption that different has negative connotations. It is essential to distinguish between assuming that having a child with a chronic condition is inherently negative and specifying which aspects of the situation are problematic (Knafl & Deatrick, 1987).

Parental concerns are often the same as those of parents whose child does not have a chronic condition. In a study about the concerns of parents of children with diabetes, the parents wanted information about diet, the child with diabetes marrying and having children, diabetes itself, care of minor illnesses, normal growth and development, and behavior management (Moyer, 1989). All of these concerns were readily addressed by the clinician. All parents worry; the extent to which a parent worries cannot be predicted from the severity of symptoms (Stein et al., 1989).

Many parents are concerned not only about the effect of a chronic condition on the family as it exists at the time of diagnosis but also about the implications for future children. A major factor is whether or not the chronic condition has a genetic component. If, for example, a family has a child with Tay-Sachs disease, the parents might choose not to have more children or might choose to use prenatal screening to assess if the fetus is affected. If the condition is genetic but not of mendelian inheritance, such as trisomy 21 with a translocation defect that might have a 3%–15% recurrence rate, the family might be more willing to risk having another child. In this case, the family can avail themselves of prenatal diagnosis. Parents who felt guilty about having a child with a genetically transmitted chronic condition will need to deal with this again if they consider having another child (Goldberg & Simmons, 1988) and later in life when their children reach childbearing age.

Family and child adaptation are interrelated. Children tend to adapt most successfully to living with a chronic condition when family functioning remains high (Grey, Boland, Sullivan-Bolyai, & Tamborlane, 1996; Hamlett, Pelligrini, & Katz, 1992; Ievers, Brown, Lambert, Hsu, & Eckman, 1998; Kell, Kliewer, Erickson, & Ohene-Frempong, 1998). Conversely, when families are not functioning optimally, families and their children tend to experience greater severity in effects related to the chronic condition. The negative effects experienced by the child are not likely to be related to the chronic condition (Drotar, 1997; Frank et al., 1998; Holden, Chimielwski, Nelson, Kager, & Foltz, 1997).

Family adaptation is likely to be influenced by a number of variables, including culture and the family's beliefs about health and illness. In a study of African American and Caucasian youths with diabetes, Auslander and colleagues (1997) found that the African American youths had significantly poorer metabolic control. The risks for African American youths was associated with single parent households and lower levels of adherence to the prescribed treatment regime. As mentioned previously, families may adopt a flexible or selective management style (Gallo & Knafl, 1998). In these situations, it is important also to evaluate the family's goals and potential barriers to working effectively with health care providers. These findings may also reflect the variation in family structure, that is the higher incidence of single parent households among African American families. In several studies on the relationship between family structure and measures of the child's health status, Silver, Stein, and Dadds (1996) and Thompson, Auslander, and White (2001) found that family structure does play a significant moderating role between the child's functional status and the child's adaptation. The effect of family structure was strongest in households where the mother lived without another related adult and when there was a stepfather in the home. These findings serve as effective reminders of the need to assess the complex family context when variations in adaptation occur. Each family should be evaluated based on their own strengths and limitations. The focus should be on the family's ability to manage the stresses related to the chronic condition rather than centering on maladaptation of the family (Clawson, 1996).

Marital Relations

Some have assumed that because the presence of a chronic condition increases the stress in a family, the rate of family dissolution is greater. On the contrary, carefully controlled studies have indicated neither differences in marital functioning nor differences in the rates of divorced or single parent families among families of children with chronic conditions (Cadman et al., 1991; Kazak, 1989a; Spaulding & Morgan, 1986). In fact, several researchers have indicated that in families of children with spina bifida, increased severity of the illness was related to higher levels of marital satisfaction for both mothers and fathers (Kazak & Clark, 1986; Martin, 1975). Although divorce is not more prevalent, tension and stress are more common than in families without a child with a chronic condition (Hobbs, Perrin, & Ireys, 1985).

It is interesting to note, that while many studies have focused on *maternal* maladjustment, Capelli and colleagues (1994) observed significant correlations between *fathers'* parenting stress and ratings of marital quality in families with a child with spina bifida. No relationships were identified for mothers. When compared with parents of healthy children, parents of children with chronic conditions were at no greater risk for psychosocial dysfunction or marital distress. Families of children with cystic fibrosis experienced greater role strain, role conflict and fewer exchanges of affection, but the parents were no more likely to experience higher levels of depression or marital dissatisfaction than families of healthy control children (Quittner, Opipari, Espelage, Carter, Eid, & Eigen, 1998). Furthermore, the negative relationship between strain and distress was mediated by the frequency and duration of social and recreational activities. Clinicians can facilitate family adjustment by encouraging family outings, recreation, and private time for spouses or partners.

Chronic Sorrow

Olshansky (1962) first described the phenomenon of *chronic sorrow* as an ongoing process that differed from grief. Olshansky's description came as a result of working with children with mental retardation. Since this early work, however, the term has been applied to many chronic conditions, both in adults and children.

Chronic sorrow refers to a pattern of sadness in response to the child's differences. Chronic sorrow is not static (Gravelle, 1997; Lowes & Lyne, 2000). Rather, the condition changes, but includes elements of permanence, with episodic surges (Hainsworth, 1996). Chronic sorrow evolves as families adapt to the full understanding of the implications of the chronic condition, including, in some cases, the possibility of the child's death (Northington, 2000). For some parents, chronic sorrow includes feelings of anger, guilt, and failure. The feelings of failure are multifaceted, and may interrelate with guilt. That relates to the inability to provide the child with a normal life.

This does not mean that the parents are always sad, or that they wish this was not their child. The lives of families in which a child has a chronic condition can be filled with happiness. They may have a tremendous appreciation of small victories. Chronic sorrow has to do with the need to redefine the parameters for judging the child's accomplishments. Families wish the affected child could have the same opportunities and experiences as other children. The triggers for exacerbations may be external, such as a child's expected date of graduation, or internal, such as an awareness that one's child will need these treatments every day for the rest of his or her life (Lindgren, Burke, Hainsworth, & Eakes, 1992). Chronic sorrow may include feelings of lack of control (Northington, 2000).

Chronic sorrow does not necessarily occur uniformly within families. Damrosch and Perry (1989) found differences between mothers and fathers. The authors stressed the need not to assess family functioning and adaptation as a unit, but also to recognize the responses of individuals within that unit. Although complex and multifaceted, chronic sorrow is not pathologic (Lowes & Lyne, 2000).

THE DYING CHILD AND THE FAMILY

While some chronic conditions improve as the child gets older, for example, certain types of asthma or juvenile arthritis, others eventually result in the child's death. This possible or probable fatality has implications for interventions with children and families. The implications and impact for survivors of a child's death, regardless of the cause, are wide-ranging and extensive.

Accepting the Possibility of Death

Most terminally ill children know that they are dying (Bluebond-Langner, 1978). Children undergoing long-term therapy to prevent or forestall death, however, are likely to suffer before their deaths. A focus on aggressive, curative care often continues even when death is inevitable; the child's symptoms are often inadequately managed (Wolfe, Grier, Klar, Levin, Ellenbogen, Salem-Schatz, Emanuel, & Weeks, 2000). Families who believe that their child is dying, in the absence of being told by physicians or other health care providers, often feel guilty and that they are giving up. A recognition of the inevitability of death not only allows for a focus on palliative care or aggressive symptom management, it also allows the patient and family the opportunity to construct an environment that the child wants. Many children choose to die at home. This has been a positive experience for most families (Collins, Stevens, & Cousens, 1998).

Another variable to be considered is the child's choices in dying. Although older data have stated that a child does not have an accurate concept of death until 11 or 12 years of age, more recent studies indicate that children as young as 5 years of age have an accurate concept of death (Mahon, 1993; Mahon, Goldberg, & Washington, 1999a). Apart from this, however, Bluebond-Langner's (1978) work with terminally ill children has indicated that these children develop a mature understanding of their illness and prognosis that is separate from their chronology. Living with a terminal illness does not mean that the child and family will constantly confront the fact of death. In fact, many of these families are similar to families in which no child is dying (Bluebond-Langner, 1996). The reality of terminal illness must be separated from the normalcy of functioning.

Caring for the child who is dying can be physically exhausting (Davies, Eng, Arcand, Collins, & Banji, 1996). The physical work occurs in addition to the emotional demands of having a child who is dying. Care must be family focused. Having this broader focus before the death provides a foundation for continuing support for the family after the death. The goal of including the family in treatment while a child is dying is to facilitate the families bereavement adaptation.

Terminally ill children of all ages may choose to forgo additional treatment meant to prolong their lives. The child may refuse surgery, dialysis, chemotherapy, or other treatment. Often the first reaction when a child asks to stop is, "he doesn't understand!" A direct and honest discussion with the child indicates that the child usually does understand. It can be helpful to use the same parameters used with adults to assess informed consent or refusal (Doig & Burgess, 2000). The child would need to demonstrate an accurate understanding of the decision, its consequences, and the risks and benefits of each option. The decision must be consistently conveyed and must be made without coercion (Mahon, Deatrick, McKnight, & Mohr, 2000). This latter is difficult because efforts are often made to talk children into entering or continuing therapies. It must be considered that the child really might choose death as less odious than continued treatments. A failure of health care providers and parents to acknowledge the child's dying results in isolation for the child, and a decreased likelihood of optimal symptom management.

After the Death

The death of a child is perhaps the most painful loss an individual can experience. Bereavement is a complex and long-term adaptation process.

Families will never be as they were before and should not be urged to get over it. The adaptation that is bereavement involves putting the child who died in a new place in the survivors' lives. There is not one specific right thing to say to support parents, but there are wrong responses. Parents should never be told "at least you have other children," "at least he was young enough so you didn't have time to know him well," "You're young. You can have more children," or worse, "I know how you feel." Even those who have experienced the death of a child will not experience the same responses.

Within families there will also be variation in response to the death of a child (Mahon & Page, 1995). Mothers are more likely to receive social support and recognition of the depth of their loss. Fathers are expected to support the mothers. This may help to explain why fathers' grief is often different from that of mothers (Hogan, 1988).

Parents are often so overwhelmed with grief it is difficult for them to support and understand the bereavement adaptation of their surviving children. Children are often reluctant to talk to their parents about their deceased sibling or matters related to the death for fear of causing their parents more pain.

Bereavement is a healthy process of adaptation, although painful and difficult. Those who interact regularly with the bereaved child, such as teachers, may not feel qualified or otherwise able to provide support for the child (Mahon, Goldberg, & Washington, 1999b). Some families benefit from counseling or support groups, although choosing not to participate is not a sign of weakness or denial; there are as many valid reasons for nonparticipation as for participating. If a referral for counseling or to a support group is made, it is essential to ascertain the therapist's or group facilitator's comfort with and qualification to address death related issues. Bereaved children should not merely be put in a loss group, in which bereaved children's issues are believed to be similar to those of children whose parents have divorced.

CONCLUSION

The family unit, varied in structure and composition, is the context of care for the child with a chronic condition. A chronic condition in a child alters the roles, expectations, and goals of all family members. Most families are able to meet the stressful demands of caring for a child with a chronic condition and even identify selected strengths in relation to the care demands. Clinicians can be instrumental in assisting the family to cope by providing family-centered care, helpful information, and by respecting the family's perspective of their situation.

REFERENCES

American Academy of Pediatrics Committee on Children with Disabilities. (2001). Counseling families who choose complementary and alternative medicine for their child with a chronic illness or disability. *Pediatrics, 107*, 598–601.

American Academy of Pediatrics Committee on School Health. (2000). Home, hospital, and other non-school-based instruction for children and adolescents who are medically unable to attend school. *Pediatrics, 106*, 1154–1155.

Amodie, N., Madrigal, A., Catala, S., Aranda-Naranjo, B., & German, V. (1997). Stress in families of HIV-positive children living in south Texas. *Psychological Reports, 81*, 1127–1133.

Auslander, W. F., Thompson, S., Dreitzer, D., White, N. H., & Santiago, J. V. (1997). Disparity in glycemic control and adherence between African-American and Caucasian youths with diabetes: Family and community contexts. *Diabetes Care, 20*, 1569–1575.

Bakewell-Sachs, S., Carlino, H., Ash, L., Thurber, F., Guyer, K., Deatrick, J. A., & Brooten, D. (2000). Home care considerations for chronic and vulnerable populations. *Nurse Practitioner Forum, 11*, 65–72.

Barbarian, O. A., Carpenter, P. J., Copeland, D. R., Dolgin, M. J., & Zeltzer, L. K. (1995). Sibling adaptation to childhood cancer collaborative study: Siblings' perceptions of the cancer experience. *Journal of Pediatric Psychology, 20*, 151–164.

Barton, S. J. (1998). Foster parents of cocaine exposed infants. *Journal of Pediatric Nursing, 13*, 104–112.

Beutler, I. F., Burr, W. R., Bahr, K. S., & Herrin, D. A. (1989). The family realm: Theoretical contributions for understanding its uniqueness. *Journal of Marriage and the Family, 51*, 805–816.

Blatt, S. D., & Simms, M. (1997). Foster care: Special children, special needs. *Contemporary Pediatrics, 14*, 109–110, 112–113, 117–118.

Bluebond-Langner, M. (1978). *The private worlds of dying children*. Princeton, NJ: Princeton University Press.

Bluebond-Langner, M. (1996). *In the shadow of illness*. Princeton, NJ: Princeton University Press.

Brodie, I., Berridge, D., & Beckett, W. (1997). Children's nursing. The health of children looked after by local authorities. *British Nursing, 6*, 386–390.

Burke, S. O., Handley-Derry, M. H., Costello, E. A., Kauffmann, E., & Dillon, M. C. (1997). Stress-point intervention for parents of repeatedly hospitalized children with chronic conditions. *Research in Nursing and Health, 20*, 475–485.

Cadman, D., Rosenbaum, P., Boyle, M., & Offord, D. R. (1991). Children with chronic illness: Family and parent demographic characteristics and psychological adjustment. *Pediatrics, 87*, 884–889.

Capelli, M., McGarth, P. J., Daniels, T., Manion, I., & Schillinger, J. (1994). Marital quality of parents of children with spina bifida: A case comparison study. *Journal of Developmental and Behavioral Pediatrics, 15*, 320–326.

Carlson, K. L. (1996). Providing health care for children in foster care: A role for advanced practice nurses. *Pediatric Nursing, 22*, 418–422.

Clawson, J. A. (1996). A child with chronic illness and the process of family adaptation. *Journal of Pediatric Nursing, 11,* 52–61.

Cohen, F. L., Nehring, W. M., Malm, K. C., & Harris, D. M. (1995). Family experiences when a child is HIV positive. *Pediatric Nursing, 21,* 248–253.

Cohen, M. H. (1993). Diagnostic closure and the spread of uncertainty. *Issues in Comprehensive Pediatric Nursing, 16,* 135–146.

Cohen, S. Y., & Wamboldt, F. S. (2000). The parent-physician relationship in pediatric asthma care. *Journal of Pediatric Psychology, 25,* 69–77.

Collins, J. J., Stevens, M. M., & Cousens, P. (1998). Home care for the dying child. A parent's perception. *Australian Family Physician, 27,* 610–614.

Coyne, I. T. (1997). Chronic illness: The importance of support for families caring for a child with cystic fibrosis. *Journal of Clinical Nursing, 6,* 121–129.

Damrosch, S. P., & Perry, L. A. (1989). Self-reported adjustment, chronic sorrow, and coping of parents of children with Down syndrome. *Nursing Research, 38,* 25–30.

Davies, B., Eng, B., Arcand, R., Collins, J., & Bhanji, N. (1996). Canuck place: A hospice for dying children. *Canadian Nurse, 92,* 22–25.

Deatrick, J., & Knafl, K. (1990). Management behaviors: Day-to-day adjustments to childhood chronic conditions. *Journal of Pediatric Nursing, 5,* 15–22.

Deatrick, J. A., Knafl, K. A., & Walsh, M. (1988). The process of parenting a child with a disability: Normalization through accommodations. *Journal of Advanced Nursing, 13,* 15–21.

Deatrick, J. A., Knafl, K. A., & Murphy-Moore, C. (1999). Clarifying the concept of normalization. *Image: The Journal of Nursing Scholarship, 31,* 209–214.

Doig, C., & Burgess, E. (2000). Withholding life-sustaining treatment: Are adolescents competent to make these decisions? *Canadian Medical Association Journal, 162,* 1585–1588.

Dokken, D. L., & Sydnor-Greenberg, N. (1998). Helping families mobilize their personal resources. *Pediatric Nursing, 24,* 66–69.

Dosa, N. P., Boeing, N. M., & Kanter, R. K. (2001). Excess risk of severe acute illness in children with chronic health conditions. *Pediatrics, 107,* 499–504.

Drotar, D. (1997). Relating parent and family functioning to the psychological adjustment of children with chronic conditions: What have we learned? What do we need to know? *Journal of Pediatric Psychology, 22,* 149–165.

Eiser, C. (1993). *Growing up with a chronic disease: The impact on children and their families.* London: Jessica Kingsley.

Feeman, D. J., & Hagen, J. W. (1990). Effects of childhood chronic illness on families. *Social Work in Health Care, 14,* 37–53.

Frank, R. G., Hagglund, K. J., Schoop, L. H., Thayer, J. F., Vieth, A. Z., Cassidy, J. T., Goldstein, D. E., Beck, N. C., Clay, D. L., Hewett, J. E., Johnson, J. C., Chaney, J. M., & Kashani, J. H. (1998). Disease and family contributors to adaptation in juvenile rheumatoid arthritis and juvenile diabetes. *Arthritis Care and Research, 11,* 166–176.

Frankel, K., & Wambolt, M. Z. (1998). Chronic childhood illness and maternal mental health—why should we care? *Journal of Asthma, 35,* 621–630.

Gallo, A. M., Breitmayer, B. J., Knafl, K. A., & Zoeller, L. H. (1992). Well siblings of children with chronic illness: Parents' reports of their psychological adjustment. *Pediatric Nursing, 18,* 23–29.

Gallo, A., & Knafl, K. (1998). Parents' reports of "tricks of the trade" for managing childhood chronic illness. *Journal of Pediatric Nursing, 3*, 93–102.

Garwick, A. W., Kohrman, C., Wolman, C., & Blum, R. W. (1998). Families' recommendations for improving services for children with chronic conditions. *Archives of Pediatric and Adolescent Medicine, 152*, 440–448.

Garwick, A. W., Patterson, J. M., Bennett, F. C., & Blum, R. W. (1998). Parents perceptions of helpful vs. unhelpful types of support in managing the care of preadolescents with chronic conditions. *Archives of Pediatric and Adolescent Medicine, 152*, 665–671.

Glazer, N. Y. (1990). The home as workshop: Women as amateur nurses and medical care providers. *Gender & Society, 4*, 479–499.

Goldberg, S., & Simmons, R. J. (1988). Chronic illness and early development, *Pediatrician, 15*, 13–20.

Gravelle, A. M. (1997). Caring for a child with a progressive illness during the complex chronic phase: Parents' experience of facing adversity. *Journal of Advanced Nursing, 25*, 738–745.

Grey, M., Boland, E. A., Yu, C., Sullivan-Bolyai, S., & Tamborlane, W. V. (1998). Personal and family factors associated with quality of life in adolescents with diabetes. *Diabetes Care, 21*, 909–914.

Hainsworth, M. A. (1996). Living with multiple sclerosis: The experience of chronic sorrow. *Journal of Neuroscience Nursing, 26*, 237–240.

Hamlett, K. W., Pelligrini, D. S., & Katz, K. S. (1992). Childhood chronic illness as a family stressor. *Journal of Pediatric Psychology, 17*, 33–47.

Hartley, B., & Fuller, C. C. (1997). Juvenile arthritis: A nursing perspective. *Journal of Pediatric Nursing, 12*, 100–109.

Hayes, V. (1997). Families and children's chronic conditions: Knowledge development and methodological considerations. *Scholarly Inquiry in Nursing Practice, 11*, 259–290.

Hill, S. A., & Zimmerman, M. K. (1995). Valiant girls and vulnerable boys: The impact of gender and race on mothers' caregiving for chronically ill children. *Journal of Marriage and the Family, 57*, 43–53.

Hobbs, N., Perrin, J. M., & Ireys, H. T. (1985). *Chronically ill children and their families.* San Francisco: Jossey-Bass.

Hogan, N. S. (1988). The effects of time on the adolescent sibling bereavement process. *Pediatric Nurse, 14*, 333–335.

Holaday, B. (1984). Challenges of rearing a chronically ill child. *Nursing Clinics of North America, 19*, 361–368.

Holden, E. W., Chmielwski, D., Nelson, C. C., Kager, V. A., & Foltz, L. (1997). Controlling for general and disease-specific effects in child and family adjustment to chronic childhood illness. *Journal of Pediatric Psychology, 22*, 15–27.

Horner, S. D. (1997). Uncertainty in mothers' care for their ill children. *Journal of Advanced Nursing, 26*, 658–663.

Hostler, S. L. (1991). Family-centered care. *Pediatric Clinics of North America, 38*, 1545–1560.

Ievers, C. E., & Drotar, D. (1996). Family and parental functioning in cystic fibrosis. *Journal of Developmental and Behavioral Pediatrics, 17*, 48–55.

Ievers, C. E., Brown, R. T., Lambert, R. G., Hsu, L., & Eckman, J. R. (1998). Family functioning and social support in the adaptation of caregivers of children with sickle cell syndromes. *Journal of Pediatric Psychology, 23*, 377–388.

Jerret, M. (1994). Parents' experience of coming to know the care of a chronically ill child. *Journal of Advanced Nursing, 19*, 1050–1056.

Jessop, D. J., Reissman, C. K., & Stein, R. E. K. (1988). Chronic childhood illness and maternal mental health. *Journal of Developmental and Behavioral Pediatrics, 9*, 147–156.

Jessop, D. J., & Stein, R. E. K. (1985). Uncertainty and its relation to the psychological correlates of chronic illness in children. *Social Science and Medicine, 20*, 993–999.

Jessop, D. J., & Stein, R. E. K. (1988). Essential concepts in the care of children with chronic illness. *Pediatrician, 15*, 5–12.

Kazak, A. E. (1989a). Families of chronically ill children: a systems and social-ecological model of adaptation and challenge. *Journal of Consulting and Clinical Psychology, 57*, 25–30.

Kazak, A. E. (1989b). Psychological issues in childhood cancer survivors. *Journal of the Association of Pediatric Oncology Nurses, 6*, 15–16.

Kazak, A. E., & Clark, M. W. (1986). Stress in families of children with myelomeningocele. *Developmental Medicine and Child Neurology, 28*.

Kell, R. S., Kliewer, W., Erickson, M. T., & Ohene-Frempong, K. (1998). Psychological adjustment of adolescents with sickle cell disease: Relations with demographic, medical, and family competence variables. *Journal of Pediatric Psychology, 23*, 301–312.

Kiburz, J. A. (1994). Perceptions and concerns of the school-age siblings of children with myelomeningocele. *Issues in Comprehensive Pediatric Nursing, 17*, 223–231.

Knafl, K., Breitmayer, B., Gallo, A., & Zoeller, L. (1996). Family responses to childhood chronic illness: Description of management styles. *Journal of Pediatric Nursing, 11*, 315–326.

Knafl, K. A., & Deatrick, J. A. (1986). How families manage chronic conditions: An analysis of the concept of normalization. *Research in Nursing and Health, 9*, 215–222.

Knafl, K. A., & Deatrick, J. A. (1987) Conceptualizing family response to a child's chronic illness or disability. *Family Relations, 36*, 300–304.

Knafl, K., Gallo, A., Breitmayer, B., Zoller, L., & Ayres, L. (1993). One approach to conceptualizing family response to illness. In S. L. Feetham, S. B. Meister, J. M. Bell, & C. L. Gillis (Eds.), *The nursing of families: Theory/research/education/ practice* (pp. 70–78). Newbury Park, CA: Sage.

Knafl, K., & Zoeller, L. (2000). Childhood chronic illness: A comparison of mothers' and fathers' experiences. *Journal of Family Nursing, 6*, 287–302.

Lindgren, C. L., Burke, M. L., Hainsworth, M. A., & Eakes, G. C. (1992). Chronic sorrow: A lifespan concept. *Scholarly Inquiry for Nursing Practice, 6*, 27–40.

Lowes, L., & Lyne, P. (2000). Your child has diabetes: Hospital or home at diagnosis? *British Journal of Nursing, 9*, 542–548.

Mahon, M. M. (1993). Children's concept of death and sibling death from trauma. *Journal of Pediatric Nursing, 8*, 335–344.

Mahon, M. M., Deatrick, J. A., McKnight, H. M., & Mohr, W. K. (2000). Discontinuing treatment in children with chronic, critical illnesses. *Nurse Practitioner Forum, 11,* 6–14.

Mahon, M. M., Goldberg, E. Z., & Washington, S. (1999a). Concept of death in a sample of Israeli children. *Death Studies, 23,* 43–59.

Mahon, M., Goldberg, R., & Washington, S. (1999b). Discussing death in the classroom: Beliefs and experiences of educators and education students. *Omega, 39,* 99–121.

Mahon, M. M., & Page, M. L. (1995). Childhood bereavement after the death of a sibling. *Holistic Nursing Practice, 9*(3), 15–26.

Martin, P. (1975). Marital breakdown in families of patients with spina bifida cystica. *Developmental Medicine and Child Neurology, 17,* 757–764.

Mastroyannopoulou, K., Stallard, P., Lewis, M., & Lenton, S. (1997). The impact of childhood non-malignant life threatening illness on parents: Gender differences and predictors of parental adjustment. *Journal of Child Psychology and Psychiatry, 38,* 823–829.

McCubbin, M. A. (1993). Family stress theory and the development of nursing knowledge about family adaptation. In S. L. Feetham, S. B. Meister, J. M. Bell, & C. L. Gillis (Eds.), *The nursing of families: Theory/research/education/practice* (pp. 46–60). Newbury Park, CA: Sage.

Meyers, A., & Weitzman, M. (1991). Pediatric HIV disease: The newest chronic illness of childhood. *Pediatric Clinics of North America, 38,* 169–191.

Morrison, L. (1997). Stress and siblings. *Paediatric Nursing, 9,* 26–27.

Moyer, F. S. (1989). Pastoral care in the hospital. *Journal of Pastoral Care, 43,* 171–183.

Northington, L. (2000). Chronic sorrow in caregivers of school age children with sickle cell disease: A grounded theory approach. *Issues in Comprehensive Pediatric Nursing, 23,* 141–154.

Olshansky, S. (1962). Chronic sorrow: A response to having a mentally defective child. *Social Casework, 43,* 190–193.

Parker, M. (1996). Families caring for chronically ill children with tuberous sclerosis complex. *Families and Community Health,* 73–84.

Patterson, J. M., Garwick, A. W., Bennett, F. C., & Blum, R. W. (1997). Social support in families of children with chronic conditions: Supportive and nonsupportive behaviors. *Journal of Developmental and Behavioral Pediatrics, 18,* 383–391.

Patterson, J., & McCubbin, H. (1983). The impact of family life events on the health of chronically ill children. *Family Relations, 32,* 255–264.

Quittner, A. L., Opipari, L. C., Espelage, D. L., Carter, B., Eid, N., & Eigen, H. (1998). Role strain in couples with and without a child with a chronic illness: Associations with marital satisfaction, intimacy, and daily mood. *Health Psychology, 17,* 112–124.

Quittner, A. L., & Opipari, L. C. (1994). Differential treatment of siblings: Interview and diary analysis comparing two family contexts. *Child Development, 65,* 800–814.

Rearson, M. A., Urban, A., Baker, L., McBride, J., Tuttle, A., & Jawad, A. (2000). Assessing parental concerns of children with diabetes. *Nurse Practitioner Forum, 11,* 20–25.

Rehm, R. S., & Franck, L. S. (2000). Long term goals and normalization strategies of children and families affected by HIV/AIDS. *Advances in Nursing Science, 23,* 69–82.

Rosenfeld, A. A., Pilowsky, D. J., Fine, P., Thorpe, M., Fein, E., Simms, M. D., Halfon, N., Irwin, M., Alfaro, J., Saletsky, R., & Nickman, S. (1997). Foster care: An update. *Journal of the American Academy of Child & Adolescent Psychiatry, 36*, 448–457.

Sheeran, T., Marvin, R. S., & Pianta, R. C. (1997). Mother's resolution of their child's diagnosis and self-reported measures of parenting stress, marital relations, and social support. *Journal of Pediatric Psychology, 22*, 197–212.

Shepard, M. P. (1992). The identification of the family system responses to the perceived impact of chronic illness which promote adaptation in a child with a chronic illness. (Doctoral dissertation, University of Pennsylvania, 1992). Dissertation Abstracts International.

Silver, E. J., Stein, R. E., & Dadds, M. R. (1996). Moderating effects of family structure on the relationship between physical and mental health in urban children with chronic conditions. *Journal of Pediatric Psychology, 21*, 43–56.

Silver, E. J., Westbrook, L. E., & Stein, R. E. (1998). Relationship of parental psychological distress to consequences of chronic health conditions in children. *Journal of Pediatric Psychology, 23*, 5–15.

Soliday, E., Kool, E., & Lande, M. B. (2000). Psychosocial adjustment in children with kidney disease. *Journal of Pediatric Psychology, 25*, 93–103.

Solnit, A., & Stark, M. (1962). Mourning the birth of a defective child. *Psychoanalytic Studies of Children, 16*, 523–536.

Spaulding, B. R., & Morgan, S. B. (1986). Spina bifida children and their parents: A population prone to family dysfunction? *Journal of Pediatric Psychology, 11*, 359–374.

Stein, A., Forrest, G. C., Wolley, H., & Baum, J. D. (1989). Life threatening illness and hospice care. *Archives of Diseases in Childhood, 64*, 697–702.

Swallow, V. M., & Jacoby, A. (2001). Mothers' coping in chronic childhood illness: The effect of presymptomatic diagnosis of vesicoureteral reflux. *Journal of Advanced Nursing, 33*, 69–78.

Thompson, S. J., Auslander, W. F., & White, N. H. (2001). Comparison of single-mother and two-parent families on metabolic control of children with diabetes. *Diabetes Care, 24*, 234–238.

Venters, M. (1981). Family coping with chronic and severe childhood illness: The case of cystic fibrosis. *Social Science and Medicine, 15a*, 289–297.

Visher, J. S., & Visher, E. B. (1995). Beyond the nuclear family: Resources and implications for pediatricians. *Pediatric Clinics of North America, 42*, 31–46.

Wallander, J. L., & Varni, J. W. (1998). Effects of pediatric chronic physical disorders on child and family adjustment. *Journal of Child Psychology and Psychiatry, 39*, 29–46.

Williams, H. A. (1993). A comparison of social support and social networks of black parents and white parents with chronically ill children. *Social Science and Medicine, 37*, 1509–1520.

Williams, P. D., Lorenzo, F. D., & Borja, M. (1993). Pediatric chronic illness: Effects on siblings and mothers. *Maternal-Child Nursing Journal, 21*, 111–121.

Wolfe, J., Grier, H. E., Klar, N., Levin, S. B., Ellenbogen, J. M., Salem-Schatz, W., Emanuel, E. J., & Weeks, J. C. (2000). Symptoms and suffering at the end of life in children with cancer. *New England Journal of Medicine, 342*, 326–333.

CHAPTER 7

Stress and Coping in Children at Risk for Medical Problems

Romy G. Engel and Barbara G. Melamed[1]

The purposes of this chapter are to (1) detail the types of stressors that may predispose children with and without chronic illness to develop health problems, (2) use developmental psychology to evaluate normative and deviant coping with medical stressors, (3) describe psychoeducational and parent or child-initiated coping which would minimize the risks, and (4) provide a schema for future research and treatment decision-making by health care professionals.

DEFINITIONS

One of the difficulties in the literature has been the lack of consensus about an operational definition of stress and coping. These terms are often used interchangeably and without respect to the developmental competence of the child. Drotar and colleagues (1989) reviewed 2 decades of the child health research and proclaimed the need for a developmental perspective to guide the focus of health promotion, also indicating where and by whom the delivery of services should occur.

[1]Acknowledgement of National Institute of Nursing Research R25-NR05098 awarded to the second author.

Several factors about chronic conditions affect the process and content of health promotion initiatives including genetic (family history of disease) and environmental factors (poverty, crowding, lack of nutrition). These factors are difficult to alter. In addition, the mental health and level of functioning of the parent are likely to affect how soon a child receives access to health care treatment, and how effectively the treatment program recommendations are implemented. For instance, many parents either cannot afford or do not completely understand the concept of continuing medication even when the symptoms have abated (e.g., antibiotic treatment). Also, access to immunizations against childhood illness is not as universal as the school requirements suggest. Once a child has been admitted to the public school system, further immunizations may not be as successful as in the preschool period. There is often excellent adherence of documentation of completed immunizations before a child starts school, however, this often lags once a child is actually a student in a system. In addition, environmentally-induced problems such as asthma or lead poisoning are difficult to change in the absence of laws protecting children. Accidental deaths are often prevented only when, for example, the absence of window guards or nonuse of seat belts are penalized. Even in these cases, new incidents of child death by inappropriate inflation of automobile air bags may confuse parents about what should constitute the proper precautions to ensure their children's safety. Furthermore, parents often do not provide children with a model of preventive habits.

To define coping as a useful construct, the taxonomy of stressors and the capacity of the individual for whom they are applicable must be clear. Thus, it is important to evaluate each child for developmental and maturational attributes, previous success in dealing with stressors, and environmental supports for healthy behaviors (including parental support, school-provided awareness and/or actual food programs, dental medical evaluations, etc.). It is also important to understand both the medical definition of adjustment to illness and the psychological advantage of acceptance of and adherence with treatment regimens.

In this chapter, research focused on issues of illness adaptation in children, from diagnosis to self-management of acute and chronic illnesses, is reviewed. A model of coping, which includes moderators and mediators of coping in response to a stressor, is presented as a guide to interventions (prevention, remediation, or teaching self-care behaviors). Illustrations of the model to preparation for surgery, adjustment to Type 1 diabetes and pediatric cancer are described. Future directions for research are also specified. In general, sampled populations included children of normal intelligence levels from families with at least one parent involved.

ASSESSMENT OF COPING

As emphasized by many child health researchers, there are few reliable and valid instruments to measure children's coping (Rudolph, Dennig, & Weisz, 1995; Ryan-Wenger, 1992; Wertlieb, Weigel, & Feldstein, 1987). It is important to assess coping to determine which coping strategies are most suitable for the numerous stressful events that children and adolescents encounter. There are several difficulties to constructing a scale to assess coping mechanisms. First, there is confusion about the difference between coping mechanisms and coping styles; the two are often used interchangeably, though they relate to different types of behavior. *Coping mechanisms*, the focus of this chapter, consist of dynamic processes, "constantly changing cognitive and behavioral efforts to manage specific internal and external demands that are appraised as taxing or exceeding the resources of the person" (Lazarus & Folkman, 1984). Implicit in this definition is the ability to alter, modify, or adjust both behaviors and thoughts in an attempt to cope with a stressor. In contrast, *coping style* is more stable over time and reflects personality characteristics. Miller and colleagues (1995) have evaluated monitoring versus blunting coping styles in children facing invasive dental procedures and finds advantages to monitoring when the stressor is controllable. Much work has been done on coping styles in adults (Suls & Wan, 1989) but little research exists in children's coping stability and outcome. In either case, the definition demands that resources of the person be considered over time. Each person's resources over time must be understood, because age as a proxy for developmental ability is deceptive if used without knowledge of conceptual level of reasoning and physical maturation or limitations imposed by illness/accident or birth defects.

It is also important not to prejudge the effectiveness of a given coping mechanism. It depends upon the purpose of a strategy, what its costs and benefits are, and how efficaciously it was used. Aldwin and Stokols (1988) have called for the examination of both positive and negative outcomes of coping on four levels: physiological, psychological, social, and cultural. In addition, long-term versus short-term effects also need to be examined.

DEFINING A TAXONOMY OF CHILDHOOD STRESSORS

Another challenge is identifying which potentially stressful situation to assess. An assessment of stressors, typically conducted by a pediatrician, nurse, social worker, child life specialist, or a psychologist, can be used to identify and evaluate multiple stressors. Table 7.1 provides a list of some of the more commonly observed stressors associated with a medical condition.

SELECTIVE REVIEW OF LITERATURE

The most common stressors studied are those associated with invasive medical procedures, for example receiving injections or undergoing dental procedures. This is a result of the frequency of such procedures and the convenience of observing a child's coping mechanism with a discrete event. These also represent frustrating and often painful events that are socially acceptable to study.

Assessing children's coping mechanisms is additionally complicated by the complexity of coping behaviors and cognitive influences. Although behaviors can be observed, actual thoughts, beliefs, or understandings can only be assessed by self-report measures. Furthermore, children's reports of their thoughts during stressful events reflect their perceptions of the coping mechanisms elicited by specific stressors. The perception may or may not be accurate. Wertlieb and colleagues (1987) referred to this as *meta-coping* and argued that understanding these perceptions is informative. Understanding the child's conceptualization of the stress and coping process is critical in engaging the child during treatment. Mischel and colleagues' (1988) findings, that the availability of alternative self-control strategies increases with age, is further evidence that the meta-coping is valid information. The differences between children's reports of their coping strategies and demonstrated actual coping techniques should be evaluated in future research. The difficulty of

TABLE 7.1 Potential Stressors Associated With Medical Condition

---

Establishing relationships with medical personnel
Coping with medical procedures associated with treatment
Coping with symptoms associated with the condition (whether acute or chronic)
Coping with possible separation from parents, other family members, and friends
Coping with social pressures, such as being labeled as ill or having a medical problem
Coping with the limitations that result from a change in lifestyle (e.g., diabetic children
     must change their diets; an asthmatic child may have to modify some physical activity)
Stress of missing school and reacclimating during the return to school
Coping with added burden facing the entire family including time and financial resources

---

assessing coping mechanisms is reflected in the vast number of categorization systems and classifications created to evaluate this strategy. These systems include: approach-avoidance (Hubert, Jay, Saltoun, & Hayes, 1988), primary versus secondary control (Band, 1990), information seeking versus information avoidance (Peterson, 1986), and control-related coping strategies (Worchel et al., 1987). This range reflects the dissatisfaction with existing assessment inventories. These researchers each created inventories that assess what they believed are the primary behaviors in a child's coping repertoire. The inventories also represent the authors' beliefs and theories about children's coping mechanisms.

The goal of this field should be to identify coping mechanisms that are most useful for a given child (including the child's cognitive development level), confronting a specific stressor, and considering prior experience with a procedure. Spirito and colleagues (1988) found that children referred for psychological evaluation due to behavioral problems used social withdrawal and distraction more frequently than nonreferred patients. These authors concluded that particular coping mechanisms, such as disengagement, can be maladaptive, however, the authors did not indicate whether there were age or disease-related stressors in the referred versus nonreferred groups.

Review of Useful Coping Tools Found in the Literature

By synthesizing a decade's worth of empirical studies based on children's coping strategies during stressors, Ryan-Wenger (1992) devised a unique categorization system. She suggested that 15 categories could be used to describe relationships between stressors and coping strategies. The categories are behaviorally grounded and have proven reliability.

Wertlieb and colleagues (1987) classified coping strategies by focus, function, and mode. *Focus* was defined as a coping behavior directed at a child's own action or the environment. *Function* is a behavior to change the problem situation, either by problem solving or emotion management. *Mode* involves information seeking, support seeking, direct actions, inhibitions of action, or intrapsychic efforts to regulate emotion. This tool has the advantage of attempting to link the stressor with the coping strategy. An even more broadly defined schema is that of Maddux and colleagues (1986), who presented a multidimensional schema relating environmental events, community, and family institutions with capability of dealing with handicapping medical conditions.

Using a single tool that assesses coping strategies of children at different ages is advantageous. It makes it possible to compare children's responses to a particular stressor at different stages of their cognitive development. The KIDCOPE was designed to assess natural and spontaneous cognitive and behavioral coping strategies of children and adolescents. Two separate age-appropriate versions were developed: one version for children 7–12 years, and another for children 13–18 years of age (Spirito, Stark, & William, 1988). The KIDCOPE can be used appropriately with a wide range of disease-related stressors; it prompts children to consider a multitude of cognitive and behavioral strategies such as problem solving, social support, emotional regulation, avoidance, and distraction. The KIDCOPE can also be used to evaluate responses to a specific stressor associated with a child's disease. The advantage of this scale is its brevity and quick assessment that can easily be integrated into clinicians' work. Such a tool is particularly useful for screening a large number of children to identify those with a limited number of coping strategies.

There have been several investigations specific to an invasive procedure or disease management. Cuthbert and Melamed (1982) developed a list of situations related to dental examinations that are likely to evoke anticipatory anxiety. The authors presented normative data on the frequency of different concerns across ages. Curry and Russ (1985) also succeeded in identifying and classifying a range of coping mechanisms that children are likely to use for dental visits. Curry and Russ linked a self-report measure and behavioral observations.

Another, more naturalistic approach is to ask children how they would help another child cope with specific situations, such as having an operation. Without assuming specific strategies, this methodology, (also employed by Ross & Ross, 1988 when classifying pain in children) Siegel's Coping Strategies Interview (CSI) (Siegel & Smith, 1991), allows a full range of responses to be described without forcing a selection from a list. This assumes that the child is comfortable with the questioner, able to conceptualize his or her own behaviors, and describe them. Younger children may be encouraged to use doll play or cartoon or puppetry to express their fears and coping strategies. (See Tables 7.2 and 7.3.)

Other approaches to pediatric coping take a more ecological point of view. In this model (Kazak, 1989) the family is viewed as a relatively homeostatic system, and a change in behavior of one family member elicits homeostatic responses from others. Thus, behaviors that seem *maladaptive* may actually be very adaptive under these circumstances. For example, we think of rigidity as a negative trait, but it may be adaptive when a rigid adherence to a medical regimen is absolutely necessary for survival (Kazak, Reber, & Snitzer, 1988).

TABLE 7.2   Age Appropriate Assessment Tools

4–7 years	Observation scales, parent report, structured interview
8–11 years	Observation scales and self-report
12 years and older	Interview, self-report, physiological measures

Families may change their strategies according to temperament characteristics of the children. For example Lumley, Abeles, Melamed, Pistone, and Johnson (1990) examined the interaction between a mother's coping behaviors and found that regardless of whether approach or avoidance coping was used it was the asynchrony of coping behaviors in the parent-child dyad that was related to distress. Thus, when both members exhibited the same style of coping there was less distress.

What really stands out in the literature is the resiliency of children. Given the proper support children bounce back and learn to cope with stressors. In fact, Wells and Schwebel (1987) found no differences in psychological disturbance or family dysfunction between chronically ill and normal children.

Appraisal of Stressor

The amount of stress associated with a stressor varies, depending on the way the child appraises the stressor. The child's stage of cognitive development also plays a role in the coping mechanisms the child uses. Therefore, the child's resources must be assessed individually taking into account conceptual level of reasoning and physical maturation or limitations imposed by illness/ accident or birth defects.

COPING STRATEGIES AS A FUNCTION OF AGE

Cognitive development has been too rarely considered in evaluations of coping mechanisms used by children and adolescents. Band (1990) argued that most researchers have virtually ignored the potential impact of developmental differences in the coping process. Wertlieb and colleagues (1987) studied two groups of children, one with an average age of 8 years and a second with an average age of 11 years, using the Children's Stress Inventory (CSI).

TABLE 7.3 Summary of Developmental Changes in Children's Use of Coping Mechanisms

Four to Seven Years of Age*
  Crying
  Screaming
  Increased physical activity
  Verbal resistance
  May need physical restraint
  Minimal use of cognitive distraction
  Use behavioral distraction
  Use primary coping

Eight to Eleven Years of Age†
  Increased use of primary coping response
  Increased use of seeking emotional support
  Decreased crying
  Decreased screaming
  Pain expressed verbally
  Muscular rigidity demonstrated
  Use cognitive distractions
  Fewer escape strategies
  Catastrophizing

Twelve to Fifteen Years of Age‡
  Increased use of secondary coping
  Decreased primary coping
  Increased muscle tension
  Decreased duration of anxious behavior
  Increased bodily control

Sixteen to Eighteen Years of Age♦
  Increased use of cognitive coping
  Increased catastrophic thought

Researchers must distinguish children's reports from those of their parents. It would be beneficial to examine whether there are differences between coping style and coping mechanisms.
*(Altshuler & Ruble, 1989; Band & Weisz, 1988; Jay, Ozolins, et al., 1983; Katz et al., 1980)
†(Altshuler & Ruble, 1989; Band, 1990; Band & Weisz, 1988; Brown et al., 1986; Katz et al., 1980)
‡(Band, 1990; Band & Weisz, 1988; Katz et al., 1980)
♦(Wertlieb et al., 1987)

They reported that emotion-management was more common among the older children, as was intrapsychic coping. This is evidence that older children use cognitive mediational control.

Curry and Russ (1985) also found significant relationships between age and coping measures used by children requiring dental work. They concluded that older children tended to implement a greater number and variety of cognitive responses in an effort to cope (Brown et al., 1986; Curry & Russ, 1985). Also, younger children sought more information than older children, and focused less on the positive aspects associated with a stressor. They found no relationship between coping mechanisms and the amount of previous dental work.

Compas and colleagues (1991) postulated several reasons for the delayed emergence of emotion-focused coping skills. First, younger children are often less aware of or able to label internal emotional states. Younger children may also fail to recognize that they have the ability to self-regulate their emotions. Last, because emotion-focused coping mechanisms are not observable in the same way as problem-focused coping, it is not possible for a child to learn this process by modeling.

Age has been consistently associated with the level of distress and coping mechanisms used during medical procedures. In fact, Jay and colleagues (1983) found age to be the strongest predictor of children's distress during bone marrow aspirations, although they did not assess the cognitive coping mechanisms of older children. This research provided evidence for a drastic decrease in children's distress scores between the ages of 6–7 years. This suggests that a cognitive development factor is operating in the experience of distress. Possibly, there is an increase in children's tolerance for pain that occurs with age.

Another possibility is that the way children appraise stress influences coping; if a child perceives the procedure to be punishment it may influence the way he or she copes (Bibace & Walsh, 1980; Perrin & Gerrity, 1981). Band (1990), too, argued that cognitive processes affect coping behaviors. There is a wealth of data suggesting that stress influences the metabolic processes influencing behavioral adherence (Hanson, Henggeler, & Burghen, 1987).

Band (1990) explored cognitive-developmental differences in coping of children with diabetes. An age effect in children's self-reports of secondary control coping has been reported by Band and Weis (1988).

Secondary control coping approaches may emerge later than primary control methods of coping. Possibly, older children can appreciate when a condition is chronic. Thus, efforts to come to terms with the fact that the disease is life long are beneficial, and may involve altering thoughts regarding the condition, rather than focusing on behaviors associated with the current state of the condition. Primary control efforts may have minimal impact on the uncontrollable nature of the disease.

Across the age groups, primary control is the most common coping mechanism employed by children with diabetes. Secondary coping, "keeping a positive attribute in order to feel better about having diabetes" proved to be a strong developmental change. A similar trend for change in coping across developmental periods was found in children with sickle cell disease (SCD) (Gil, Thompson, Keith, TotaFaucette, Noll, & Kinney, 1993). In a longitudinal study of children and adolescents with SCD and their parents, coping attempts were contrasted with passive adherence and negative thinking. The status of the child's illness was reassessed 9 months later. Children with SCD can anticipate many painful episodes, although the onset of pain is not predictable and the duration is highly variable. Using the Coping Strategies Questionnaire, Rosenstiel and Keefe (1983) found reliable pain coping strategies that were significantly related to adjustment during painful episodes. Children with higher numbers of coping attempts were more active and required less frequent health care services than children who had more negative thinking and passive adherence. Younger children tended to be more stable in their use of coping over time. Older children varied more, particularly in increase or decrease of negative thinking. The increase in negative thinking was associated with more health care visits, whereas the decrease in negative thinking was related to fewer. In that symptom reporting is often used by parents to decide when the children need health care services, this is not surprising. It may even be that the older children correctly identify the onset of a pain episode because of repeated previous experiences. They may have come to rely more on health care services for their pain management (Table 7.3).

LIMITATIONS AND GAPS IN THE LITERATURE

A review of the literature in the field of children's ability to cope with medical stressors reveals a lack of research on stressors other than those related to painful medical procedures. The advantage of examining coping mechanisms in this context is the convenience of assessing a discrete event. Other stressors such as depression with a diagnosis of a chronic illness or hospitalization may require more longer-term coping mechanisms.

There is a lack of research on coping over time. Changes in coping mechanisms over the course of an illness are not well documented (Spirito et al., 1988). Several researchers have sought to establish this temporal relationship (Jay et al., 1983); changes in coping mechanisms and level of stress are hypothesized to occur over time. These researchers examined whether a habituation phenomenon occurred with children and adolescents undergoing multiple bone marrow aspirations (BMAs). They found that children do habituate over time and with experiences. Interestingly, a stronger habituation effect was found for children 2–7 years of age and a modest habituation effect for the two older groups. For habituation to occur in the youngest group took time and a significant amount of exposure: 12 BMA procedures in 2 years for children younger than age 7. For older children, habituation took less time.

Comparisons of coping mechanisms across types of stressors is often inappropriate, since, for example, the pain of the anesthetic injection for dental treatment is far less traumatic than bone marrow aspirations. Furthermore, the contexts of these situations differ greatly.

FLEXIBILITY IN COPING MECHANISMS

It has often been pointed out that not only must the effective coping repertoire exist, but also the child must be aware of when and how to use these strategies effectively. Children can learn how to compensate for, or even hide, behaviors that can be injurious. Children can also, then, learn positive compensatory behaviors. Certain monitoring techniques can be used to teach a child when a change will be effective in promoting stability of the physiology in light of an illness.

DEVELOPING A LINKAGE MODEL

Enough data do exist from the current review to postulate different pathways that would allow formulation of strategies for children's coping. Ideally, such a model could be used with children across diagnoses or procedures. Such a model provided by Rudolph, Dennig, and Weisz (1995) illustrates the usefulness for decision making. They focus on the moderator and mediator variables involved in the coping process. They describe situation-specific

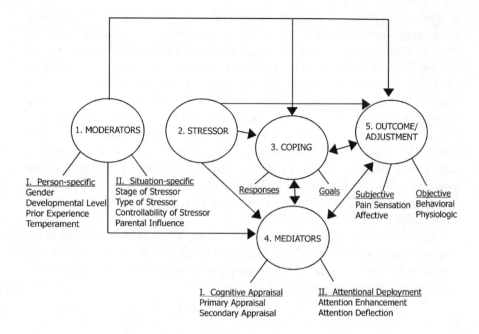

FIGURE 7.1   Model of variables involved in the coping process.

and person-specific variables (see Figure 7.1). In looking at coping goals and stress outcomes they carefully discuss the fact that it may be that poor coping leads to maladaptive behaviors and vice-versa. The nature of the stress to be overcome, the length of time (effort) in maintaining the coping strategy, and the developmental cognitive abilities to be accessed given the age of the child must also be considered.

The rationale underlying provision of information is that unexpected stress is more anxiety provoking and more difficult to cope with than anticipated or predictable stress. Therefore, we must view the child's previous experience in coping. Optimal interventions with children require information about the child's illness, previous experiences, developmental level, and concurrent stressors in the family. This information can be gathered by reports obtained from the child (self-reports, behavioral observations, checklists), parental knowledge (questionnaire, interview, child's perception of involvement) and coordination, and input from the health care professionals. A multidisciplinary team is ideal when working with children and families. Any intervention must be reevaluated (1) when the child reaches a higher level of cognitive functioning and can take a more self-management role, (2) the health of family members changes, (3) other family stressors occur, (4) if the disease remits and adherence is the main focus, (5) if access to health care changes, and (6) if technological advances change the method of diagnosis or treatment regimen.

Spirito and colleagues (1995) developed a very useful database by their study of 177 children with various chronic illnesses. Some coping strategies were used equally across illness-related stressors. Others, such as distraction, blaming, and emotional regulation, varied by stressor. Along with the naturalistic field work of Siegel and Smith (1991) these authors suggested that evaluation of coping skills, and whether they are adaptive in altering, for example, the course of disease or pain tolerance, can best be understood within the context of a cognitive developmental model. In addition, previous experiences, beliefs about the ability to manage the stressors, and additional family factors determine the coping strategies that will be most effective at a given point in time. It is understood that change is a necessary part of the optimal use of such strategies at times of increased stress, higher cognitive functioning, or high demanding environmental situations (i.e., marriage, relocation, job loss, etc.). Family records along with the medical records allow collaboration with the family and between professionals about specifics of and changes in care.

IMPLICATIONS FOR INTERVENTION

Jay (1988) outlines the various methods that have been involved with helping children cope. She includes puppets, modeling films, coloring books, and further, gives examples of when hypnosis, behavior therapy, and cognitive behavioral approaches would be indicated.

In order to demonstrate the usefulness of a model of linking stressors coping and outcomes, we provide examples from the literature of one acute stressor hospital preparation. By age 7 years more than 50% of all children would be likely to have encountered an emergency room or overnight stay in a hospital. The second part of this section demonstrates how knowing about developmental periods will facilitate consideration of crucial risk factors. Type 1 diabetes and cancer in childhood are used for illustrative purposes. When a child has diabetes, the child and family must learn to live with a complex medical regimen including diet, behavior, and injection and regulation of insulin. The diagnosis of cancer in childhood is stressful in terms of the devastation of the diagnosis. Although increasing numbers of children are surviving, there remain many issues related to the pain that is almost uniformly a part of diagnosis and treatment.

Preparation for Hospitalization and Acute Invasive Procedures

Estimates of behavioral disturbances range from 10–92% in children who experience hospitalization.These include regressive behavior (such as increased dependency, loss of toilet training), increased fears, and sleep and eating disturbances. Ten to thirty-five percent of children develop serious long-term disturbances. Psychological preparation can, however, influence the course of illness and responses to stress (Visintainer & Wolfer, 1975; Wolfer & Visintainer, 1975; Wolfer & Visintainer, 1979).

Several factors influence coping. Researchers (Melamed & Ridley-Johnson, 1988) have demonstrated the relationship of coping and improved rate of healing, reduction of discomfort, control of pain, and decreased nausea, vomiting, blood pressure, and heart rate. What is it that children associate with invasive procedures that is frightening and how does this differ in different stages of development? The uncertainty of outcome, fear of pain, and loss of control underlie much of the anxiety children experience when confronted with unknown medical procedures. Even a first haircut can be frightening for a toddler: uncertainty, fear, and loss of control exist. In very young children separation from the primary caretaker is a major cause of anxiety. In those approaching puberty, loss of social contact, fear of body harm, and fear of ridicule for being different are more likely to be of concern. Children bring with them to any event the history of similar experiences and their successes and failures in dealing with those challenges. In children who have been overprotected, the lack of development of self-control over the management of stress may result from adults' attempts to protect the child. Thus, the child is without a repertoire of behaviors for handling unpreventable and noxious events.

Many coping behaviors can be taught; the strategies should be specific to the procedure the child must undergo. For example, if a child must receive an injection, it may be sufficient to employ their natural interests and use distraction with other objects (TV, music, ceiling tiles) during the event. Most procedures are more complex, and might include separation from loved ones, strange sights and sounds, unpleasant smells, and the presence of strange people, instruments, and medications.

Children's coping is affected by preparation; the timing of this preparation is critical. Children aged 7 and younger can be frightened and react more disruptively if they are prepared too early (Melamed, Meyer, Gee, & Soule, 1986). Older children may be able to reinvoke coping strategies previously successfully used if they are instructed about what the upcoming procedures will entail. Here again, it is most important to understand how each child processes and makes use of information. In many cases, the use of filmed modeling, which relies on a child similar in age and appearance to the child being prepared, is successful in stimulating coping responses (Melamed & Siegel, 1975). In this case, the child receives information about what to expect and observes strategies being used to deal with these events. Thus, the experience is normalized, the child is reinforced for practicing these strategies prior to undergoing the procedure. The expectation for control is bolstered by actually having a repertoire of behaviors to use.

Patient variables (e.g., age, prehospital experience, previous coping responses) are brought to the current situation. Preparation related to treatment variables, then, focuses on reducing anxiety, providing information, support, behavioral rehearsal, or in the case of avoidant children, systematic desensitization or participant modeling. When the patient variables are ignored there may be a sensitization effect. Children with few prior experiences need information and models of coping even more than children who have developed effective coping styles. Younger children (< 7 years) with a previous negative hospital experience, who were prepared using a filmed model of what to expect, were more disruptive and anxious (Melamed et al., 1983). When a stressor is unpredictable it may be better to focus attention away from it rather than building up anticipatory anxiety.

Managing Cancer Diagnosis and Treatment

A major stressor for children with cancer is the pain of repeated bone marrow aspirations and lumbar punctures necessary to determine the progress of the illness and to identify optimal treatments (see chapter 4). It is critical to define both psychological and physical pain in the construct of behavioral distress (Katz, Kellerman, & Siegel, 1980), and to consider verbal, behavioral, and physiological expressions of discomfort. Adult assessment measures tend to rely on verbal reports and are not appropriate for use with children. For very young children, tools to assess pain include pictorial representations of affect (FACES). Intensity is usually related to a thermometer or a visual analogue scale (Hicks, von Baeyer, Spafford, vanKorlaar, & Goodenough,

2001). Color has been used to assess the intensity of the child's fear or pain. For very young children pain-induced vocalization and movement actographs have been used, but standardization is not yet established. Hester (1979) found that the use of poker chips from 1–4 ("none" to "most hurt possible") has validity with younger children. Rape and Bush (1994) concluded that few studies of the efficacy of hypnosis and cognitive-behavioral packages in preparing pediatric oncology patients considered the moderating effect of developmental age.

Behavioral observation methods have been used successfully with children; they are especially valuable because they circumvent the problems of self-report measures. Behavioral observation does not rely on the child's under-standing or ability to verbalize experiences. Several groups of researchers have attempted to quantify pediatric cancer patients' pain/discomfort during bone marrow aspirations and lumbar punctures (Jay et al., 1983; Katz et al., 1980; LeBaron & Zeltzer, 1984). These scales, including the Procedural Behavior Rating Scale and the Observation Scale of Behavioral Distress, have established interrater reliabilities and have correlated well with anxiety and pain ratings from independent scales. The Procedure Rating Checklist correlates significantly with observation checklists and self-reports. Again, developmental norms must be applied. Katz and colleagues (1980) demon-strated that previous experience interacts with developmental age to determine the sensitivity of the child on these scales. Lavigne, Schulein, and Hahn (1986) presented an excellent review of cognitive changes in pain perception of the development from younger to older children.

Managing Type 1 Diabetes: Conditions Triggering Loss of Metabolic Control

The development of Type 1 diabetes unfolds as the pancreas fails to develop the insulin-regulating mechanism that allows most people to maintain blood glucose stability. Monitoring of blood glucose levels is an essential component of managing a child's diabetes (see chapter 2).

To understand the role of cognitive development in children's coping with diabetes, Band (1990) and Band and Weisz (1988) asked children of different ages to rate their perceptions of control and coping efficacy, and to describe their coping strategies across a broad range of diabetes specific stresses including: staying well, diet, insulin reactions, daily glucose, and hemoglobin A_{1c} testing, and diet. She related their developmental stage with strategies and diabetes adjustment measures. The children with less cognitive maturity tended to rely more on primary types of instrumental and social-emotional strategies. Older children were more likely to engage in efforts to control the conditions by such actions as taking their blood sugar levels, finding meaning (reinterpretation) in diet restrictions, and by keeping a positive attitude. As children reached adolescence, there was a sense that one must cope with the chronic nature of the disorder. Johnson and Rosenbloom (1982) found that adolescents had difficulty with the management regimen, possibly because of a need for self-regulation and autonomy. Researchers doing a longitudinal study (Goldston et al., 1995) found that pervasive noncompliance in adolescents with diabetes was related to severity of life events as recorded by the parents.

In a study conducted at a summer camp (Olson, Johansen, Powers, Pope, & Klein, 1993), more similarities than differences were found across chronic illnesses on the types of coping strategies used. When compared with a healthy public school population, it was found that coping within the chronic illness groups (asthma, diabetes, juvenile rheumatoid arthritis) varied by age and gender. The use of cognitive coping strategies increased with age; however, there were no significant differences between the chronic illness and control groups. The frequency of use of cognitive coping increased with age in healthy and ill children. Children tended to use different coping strategies with different types of stressors.

Family Adaptation

It is critical not only to look at the individual coping with stress of illness but to focus on parental adaptation to illness. It is important to remember that non-ill siblings are also challenged and may have to take on additional roles and often suffer the consequence of reduced parental attention. One central research issue is how to measure family adaptation. The Family Adaptation and Cohesion and the Family Crisis Oriented Personal Evaluation Scales Scale (Olson et al., 1985) are typically used to look in-depth at the types of changes families experience during the course of a child's illness. A research scale called the Maternal Worry Scale (DeVet & Ireys, 1998) has demonstrated good internal reliability and validity and may be a sensitive measure of maternal anxiety as it is related to having a sick child. Its use was sensitive to developmental change with mothers' report of internalizing and externalizing behaviors of their older children being related to greater worry.

One problem has been a lack of definition in what is an adaptive family. Weiss, Marvin, and Pianta (1997) provided a systems analysis in their ethnographic approach to describing families caring for children with cerebral palsy. They identified three types of adjustment patterns: the traditional pattern where the mother is solely responsible for childcare, the team pattern where both parents are highly active in child care, and the extended family pattern where childcare is spread out across biologically related individuals. A formal support pattern is a strategy of distributing a very significant amount of responsibility for childcare to professional and educational providers. Each of these patterns of family care led to good school and home adjustment of the child.

Empowerment

Investigators have used the Family Empowerment Scale (Koren et al., 1997) and found that there was further validation of the empowerment concept. It was also found that a higher sense of parental empowerment is significantly related to children's better adherence to treatment, including metabolic control. Whereas, most previous studies have focused on the negative aspects of mothers' coping, one study (Florian & Elad, 1998) defined the construct of *empowerment* to describe the ongoing capacity of individuals or groups to act on their own behalf to achieve a greater measure of control over their lives and destinies. Jones, Garlow, Turnbull, and Barber (1996) defined five ideas in relation to the construct of empowerment: (1) perceived control and efficacy over the course of life events, (2) effectiveness influencing life conditions through problem-solving skills, coping strategies, and effective use of resources, (3) family-professional partnerships, (4) community participation, including leadership in organizations, and (5) situational and temporal variability. Empowerment takes different forms in divergent contexts, differs across individuals in the same context, and may change over time for the same individual.

Observational Methodology

An observational approach taken by Hauser and colleagues (Hauser, DiPlacido, Jacobsen, Willett, & Cole, 1993) has revealed many features of families dealing with the onset of insulin-dependent diabetes in comparison with families facing an acute illness. They examined the micro level, looking in detail at how aspects of family communication and interaction may be linked with child or adolescent vulnerability and resilience. The unit of analysis here was the individual family member in relation to and in interaction with other members of the family. Their descriptions of coping strategies have been operationally defined. Interview material is audiotaped, and trained raters code the verbal statements of family members into categories of appraisal-focused (cognitive processes), problem-focused (behavioral efforts), and emotion management coping strategies (strategies that deal with emotional regulation of problem feelings). Family cohesiveness is addressed by evaluating specific statements of how individual family members see the unit functioning. These studies are longitudinal so they will yield important information about changes over the course of development of the family and the adolescent.

Preliminary findings on 42 diabetic families and 37 acute illness families suggest that mothers of diabetics describe their families as seeking support, pursuing alternative rewards, and trying out new responses compared to acute illness families, who see their families as being more self-reliant and operating as a consensual unit (e.g., "we are all in this together" view). Fathers also describe the acute illness families as pursuing alternative rewards, seeking support and trying out new responses. They do not see their families as more self-reliant than those with acute illness families. The adolescents in diabetic families characterized their families as being less involved in seeking information about their current difficulties. Regarding emotion-management strategies, the diabetic families expressed their feelings to others outside the family and described more impulsive expressions of their feelings than those parents of children with acute illnesses. The diabetic youngsters were less likely to minimize their awareness of their own and other family members' feelings.

It is evident from the research studies of this group of investigators (e.g., Hauser, Vieyra, Jacobson, & Wertlieb, 1989) that the three domains of protective factors—personality, social, and familial—frequently interact as determinants of resilient developmental outcomes.

Garmezy (1984) detailed a series of possibilities regarding how personal attributes and stressful events may interact to determine the quality of adaptation. Stress factors and personal attributes may combine additively in the prediction of outcome. Stress (if not excessive) may enhance competence; this is the *challenge* model. Or, an alternative perspective suggests that personal attributes may modulate, buffer, or exacerbate the impact of stress.

Hauser and colleagues (1986) looked at transactional father-child relationships in IDDM, using direct observation codes; they found differential patterns of interaction for mothers and fathers. Whereas mothers engaged in more enabling behaviors toward their children (e.g., empathy, assurance, problem solving), fathers engaged in more constraining behaviors (e.g., devaluation, indifference, judging critically).

ETHNIC, RACIAL, AND GENDER EFFECTS ON COPING

There have been few studies that have specifically focused on racial or religious differences experienced by families with sick children. One study (Williams, Lorenzo, & Borja, 1993) of African American and European American parents examined the characteristics of social networks and provision of support in families with a child who has cancer; it found that, whereas social support appears to buffer distress, the types of social support varied. African American parents described support as instrumental actions, whereas European Americans focused more on affective and emotional support. It was noted in this study that the European American families had support networks twice as large as African Americans, although the African American parents perceived their networks as being more supportive. Another study (Rehm, 2000) looked specifically at Mexican Americans' religiosity as an influence on coping with disease; despite the feeling that God is Supreme, there was active coping by the family and collaboration with medical avenues.

Family cohesion appears to have a differential impact on African American boys and girls with sickle cell disease (SCD) (Hurtig, Koepke, & Park, 1989). Girls tend to become more aggressive with parental conflict, whereas low cohesiveness leads to increased somatic, uncommunicative, and schizoid problems in boys.

PROSPECTIVE RESEARCH DESIGN

One of the more positive changes in research on parenting ill children has been the adoption of prospective research designs, which follow the family coping across the various phases of illness. Frank, Thayer, Hagglund, et al. (1998), using growth analyses, looked at single family adaptation patterns to two diseases, juvenile rheumatoid arthritis (JRA) and Type 1 diabetes (IDDM). They found that across families, maternal dysphoria was highest at time of diagnosis. The parents of children with JRA were more likely to maintain distress and report difficulty in control of the illness than parents of children with IDDM or healthy children (adaptation or maturation over time). It could be that physical disability, which often accompanies JRA, may be more apparent than the life-threatening aspects of IDDM. In evaluating the importance of timing of social support (as it may reduce anxiety in parents) following transplant procedures, Rodrigue, MacNaughten, Hoffman III, Graham-Pole, Andres, Novak, and Fennell (1997) revealed that 6 months following the procedure the extended family had reduced or withdrawn their support. It was just at this time when anxiety increased due to the arrival of medical bills and compliance problems with use of drugs to prevent rejection.

In a longitudinal 4-year study of adolescents with IDDM, Seiffge-Krenke (1998) evaluated the effects of a highly structured climate in families of adolescents and used a control group of healthy children. She found that those parents with a sick child reported on the average a significantly worse emotional climate, but a higher amount of structure and organization. However, family environment did not predict metabolic control over the course of time. The findings that adolescents with diabetes and their parents have a family climate characterized by a high amount of structure, organization, control, and achievement orientation are consistent with findings of enmeshed patterns of interaction in families dealing with Type 1 diabetes (Hauser & Solomon, 1985). In addition, Hanson et al. (1995) similarly found a lack of direct effects of family climate on metabolic control but an indirect effect through positive adherence to the medical regimen. Thus, it seems that, in order to improve compliance, close monitoring by parents is desirable.

PREADOLESCENT VULNERABILITY

Several studies have focused on preadolescent children, as this is a unique developmental period in which autonomy and independence compete with parents' concerns for controlling the illness regimen. In addition, change in hormones makes regulation of disease processes more difficult even with excellent compliance. Johnson and her colleagues (2000) found poorer metabolic control in preadolescents. Goldston and colleagues (1995) found that pervasive noncompliance mediated metabolic control in adolescents particularly where there was a perceived intensification of stressful life events.

A study using a wide collection of self-report measures on adolescents and their parents (Kell, Kliewer, Erikson, & Ohene-Frempong, 1998) found that, after controlling for disease severity, sociodemographic, and medical variables, scores on the Self-Report Family Inventory (SFI) revealed that higher levels of family competence were associated with fewer behavioral and emotional problems. Interestingly, the influence was greater for younger adolescents and in predicting internalizing problems and somatic complaints among girls. Again, this design was correlational, so that no causal relations can be concluded.

A study of preadolescents who had been living with chronic illnesses was conducted in which parents were asked what were helpful versus unhelpful types of support. Garwick, Patterson, Bennett, and Blum (1998) found that both mothers and fathers reported that other family members were the primary source of helpful emotional and tangible support, whereas health care providers were the primary source of helpful informational support. They held in-depth in-home evaluations on two occasions 1 year apart. They found that fathers reported more helpful emotional and informational support from family members 1 year later. Regarding unsupportive behaviors, one third attributed them to health care providers and another third to extended family members. The types of things that were unhelpful from health care providers included insensitivity, rudeness, a negative attitude toward the child or family, inadequate information about the child's condition or care, inadequate services or referrals. Approximately half were related to communication problems. Extended family members were cited as having inadequate contact or involvement with the child or family, provided inadequate emotional support, made insensitive or invasive comments, or blamed the parents for the child's condition. Acquaintances, neighbors, and community persons were faulted for insensitive comments and questions, lack of understanding, and withdrawal of friendship. School providers were also cited for inadequate services, insensitivity to the child's needs, and lacking knowledge about a child's condition. It is important to assess social support within the context of the setting in which it is perceived given that parents have different experiences of what they need from different individuals. Parents appear to expect particular types of support from specific sources.

PRACTICAL INFORMATION ABOUT PARENTING ILL CHILDREN

There are at least 10 strategies that would contribute to enhancing resilience for a family with an ill child:

(1) Balancing the illness with other family needs. Roles, that is, status and behavioral expectations, are relatively well defined in families. Therefore, if a child needs special attention or is hospitalized, there must be a shift in roles. Attention to sibling needs by including extended family during crisis periods can alleviate some of the tension. Having outside paid help to shop, clean, and do other chores will free up time for accomplishing basic family commitments to each other.

(2) Maintaining clear family boundaries. During an illness crises, the extended family may assist with normal chores or usurp the role of the parents

in disciplining the children. It is important to make it clear that the needs will change over the course of the child's illness.

(3)   Developing communication competence. Learning how to talk to the physicians about their concerns and how to help the child communicate their disability to others.

(4)   Attributing positive meanings to the situation. Some families become closer when adversity of illness occurs as they show that the family can maintain its coherence during crises.

(5)   Maintaining family flexibility; less rigidity at who does what.

(6)   Maintaining a commitment to the family as a unity.

(7)   Engaging in active coping efforts.

(8)   Modeling good coping efforts and facilitating approach-oriented problem solving.

(9)   Maintaining social integration (e.g., participation in church, community, and school); and

(10)   Developing collaborative relationships with professionals.

SUMMARY AND CONCLUSIONS

Many factors affect children's coping. Coping strategies are an important part of health and disease management. Standardized tools are needed to evaluate coping strategies in the context of a wide range of stressors and personal resources. Cognitive development and disease factors converge to make each child's coping unique. Family factors and changes in dynamic relationships must be considered in evaluating resources and potential problems. The emotional well-being of the child is crucial. Children need to develop social networks and peer affiliations. The red flags that indicate a child's difficulty in moving through the normal sequence of adjustment should lead to intervention for development of greater self-management strategies for coping with the stressors. A serious gap in the literature is the lack of well-documented changes in coping mechanisms over the course of an illness.

Interventions need to consider the task required to adapt to the stressors. Whether or not this is ongoing in chronic illness management or short-term in treatment or diagnosis is important in defining the type of intervention and who should administer it.

The need for development of assessment tools for both the child and family interactions is critical in predicting difficulties and setting forth prevention interventions. More prospective research is indicated in following up these children and evaluating the strength of these predictors. This chapter sets forth a functional analyses by which tasks can be conceptualized as to necessary skills in parenting chronically ill children and evaluating the child's resources for resilience.

REFERENCES

Altshuler, J. L., & Ruble, D. N. (1989). Developmental changes in children's awareness of strategies for coping with uncontrollable stress. *Child Development, 60,* 1337–1349.

Aldwin, C., & Stokols, D. (1988). The effects of environmental change on individuals and groups: Some neglected issues in stress research. *Journal of Environmental Psychology, 8,* 57–75.

Band, E. B. (1990). Children's coping with diabetes: Understanding the role of cognitive development. *Journal of Pediatric Psychology, 15,* 27–41.

Band, E. B., & Weisz, J. R. (1988). How to feel better when it feels bad: Children's perspectives on coping with every-day stress. *Developmental Psychology, 24*(2), 247–253.

Bibace, R., & Walsh, M. E. (1980). Development of children's concepts of illness. *Pediatrics, 66*(6), 912–917.

Boyce, W. T., & Jemerin, J. M. (1990). Psychobiological differences in childhood stress response. I. Patterns of illness and susceptibility. *Developmental and Behavioral Pediatrics, 11*(2), 86–94.

Brown, J. M., O'Keefe, J., Sanders, S. H., & Baker, B. (1986). Developmental changes in children's cognition to stressful and painful situations. *Journal of Pediatric Psychology, 11*(3), 343–357.

Compas, B. E., Banez, G. A., Malcarne, V., & Worsham, N. (1991). Perceived control and coping with stress: A developmental perspective. *Journal of Social Issues, 47*(4), 23–34.

Curry, S. L., & Russ, S. W. (1985). Identifying coping strategies in children. *Journal of Clinical Child Psychology, 14*(1), 61–69.

Cuthbert, M. I., & Melamed, B. G. (1982). A screening device: Children at risk for dental fears and management problems. *Journal of Dentistry for Children, 49,* 432–436.

DeVet, K. A., & Ireys, H. T. (1998). Psychometric properties of the maternal worry scale for children with chronic illness *Journal of Pediatric Psychology, 23,* 257–266.

Drotar, D., Johnson, S. B., Iannotti, R., Krasnegor, N., Matthews, K. A., Melamed, B. G., Millstein, S., Peterson, R. A., Popiel, D., & Routh, D. K. (1989). Child health psychology. *Health Psychology, 8*(6), 781–784.

Florian, V., & Elad, D. (1998). The impact of mothers' sense of empowerment on the metabolic control of their children with juvenile diabetes. *Journal of Pediatric Psychology, 23,* 239–247.

Frank, R. G., Thayer, J. F., Hagglund, K. J., Vieth, A. Z., Schopp, L. H., Beck, N. C., Kashani, J. H., Goldstein, D. E., Cassidy, J. T., Clay, D. L., Chaney, J. M., Hewett, J. E., & Johnson, J. C. (1998). Trajectories of adaptation in pediatric chronic illness:

The importance of the individual. *Journal of Consulting and Clinical Psychology, 66,* 521–532.

Garmezy, N. (1984). Stress-resistant children: The search for protective factors. In J. E. Stevenson (Ed.), *Recent research in developmental psychopathology.* Journal of Child Psychology and Psychiatry Book Supplement, No. 4. Oxford: Pergamon Press.

Garwick, A., Patterson, J., Bennett, F., & Blum, R. (1998). Parents' perceptions of helpful versus unhelpful types of support in managing the care of preadolescents with chronic conditions. *Archives of Pediatric Adolescent Medicine, 152,* 665–671.

Gil, K., Thompson, R., Keith, B., TotaFaucette, M., Noll, S., & Kinney, T. (1993). Sickle cell disease pain in children and adolescents: Changes in pain frequency and coping strategies over time. *Journal of Pediatric Psychology, 18*(5), 621–637.

Goldston, D. B., Kovacs, M., Obrosky, D. S., & Iyengar, S. (1995). A longitudinal study of life events and metabolic control among youths with insulin-dependent diabetes mellitus. *Health Psychology, 14,* 409–414.

Hanson, C., DeGuire, M., Schinkel, A., & Kolterman, O. (1995). Empirical validation for a family-centered model of care. *Diabetes Care, 10,* 1347–1356.

Hanson, C. L., Henggeler, S. W., & Burghen, G. A. (1987). Social competence and parent support as mediators of the link between stress and metabolic control in adolescents with insulin-dependent diabetes mellitus. *Journal of Consulting and Clinical Psychology, 55,* 529–533.

Hauser, S., Jacobson, D., Wertlieb, B., et al. (1986). Children with recently diagnosed diabetes: Interactions with their families. *Health Psychology, 5,* 273–296.

Hauser, S., & Solomon, M. (1985). Coping with diabetes: Views from the family. In P. I. Ahmed & N. Ahmed (Eds.), *Coping with juvenile diabetes* (pp. 234–266). Springfield, IL: Thomas.

Hauser, S. T., DiPlacido, J., Jacobsen, A. M., Willett, J., & Cole, C. (1993). *Journal of Adolescence, 16*(3), 305–329.

Hauser, S., Vierya, M., Jacobson, A., & Wertlieb, D. (1989). Family aspects of vulnerability and resilience in adolescence: A theoretical perspective. In T. F. Dugan & R. Coles (Eds.), *The child in our times: Studies in the development of resiliency.* New York: Brunner/Mazel, Publishers.

Hester, N. K. (1979). The preoperational child's reaction to immunization. *Nursing Research, 28,* 250–254.

Hicks, L. L., vonBaeyer, C. L., Spafford, P. A., vanKorlaar, I., & Goodenough, B. (2001). The FACES Pain Scale—Revised: Toward a common metric in pediatric pain measurement. *Pain, 93*(2), 173–183.

Hubert, N., Jay, S., Saltoun, M., & Hayes, M. (1988). Approach-avoidance and distress in children undergoing preparation for painful medical procedures. *Journal of Clinical Child Psychology, 17*(3), 194–202.

Hurtig, A. L., Koepke, D., & Park, K. B. (1989). Relation between severity of chronic illness and adjustment in children and adolescents with sickle cell disease. *Journal of Pediatric Psychology, 14,* 117–132.

Jay, S. (1988). Invasive medical procedures: Psychological intervention and assessment. In D. Routh (Ed.), *Handbook of pediatric psychology* (pp. 401–426). New York: Guilford Press.

Jay, S., Ozolin, M., Elliot, C., & Caldwell, S. (1983). Assessment of children's distress during painful medical procedures. *Health Psychology, 2,* 133–148.

Johnson, S. B., Perwien, A. R., & Silverstein, J. H. (2000). Response to hypo- and hyperglycemia in adolescents with type 1 diabetes. *Journal of Pediatric Psychology, 25*(3), 171–178.

Johnson, S. B., & Rosenbloom, A. L. (1982). Behavioral aspects of diabetes mellitus in childhood and adolescence. *Psychiatric Clinics of North American, 5*(2), 357–369.

Jones, T., Garlow, J., Turnbull, H., Rutherford, III, & Barber, P. (1996). Family empowerment in a family support program. In G. Singer & L. Powers (Eds.), *Redefining family support: Innovations in public-private partnerships* (Vol. 1). Baltimore, MD: Brookes Publishing Co.

Katz, E., Kellerman, J., & Siegel, S. E. (1980). Behavioral distress in children with cancer undergoing medical procedures: Developmental considerations. *Journal of Consulting and Clinical Psychology, 48,* 356–365.

Kazak, A. (1989). Families of chronically ill children: A systems and social-ecological model of adaptation and change. *Journal of Consulting and Clinical Psychology, 57,* 25–30.

Kazak, A., Reber, M. I., & Snitzer, L. (1988). Childhood chronic disease and family functioning: A study of phebylketonuria. *Pediatrics, 81,* 224–230.

Kell, R. S., Kliewer, W., Eriksonh, M. T., & Ohene-Frempong, K. (1998). Psychological adjustment of adolescents with sickle cell disease: Relations with demographic, medical, and family competence variables. *Journal of Pediatric Psychology, 23,* 301–312.

Koren, P. E., DeChillo, N., Friesen, B. J., Singh, N., Curtis, W., Ellis, C., Wechsler, H., Best, A., & Cohen, R. (1997). Empowerment status of families whose children have serious emotional disturbance and attention-deficit/hyperactivity disorder. *Journal of Emotional and Behavioral Disorders, 5,* 223–229.

Lavigne, J., Schulein, M., & Hahn, Y. (1986). Psychological aspects of painful medical conditions in children. Developmental aspects and assessment. *Pain, 27,* 133–146.

Lazarus, R. S., & Folkman, S. (1984). *Stress, appraisal, and coping.* New York: Springer.

LeBaron, S., & Zeltzer, L. (1984). Assessment of acute pain and anxiety in children and adolescents by self-reports, observer reports, and a behavior checklist. *Journal of Consulting and Clinical Psychology, 52,* 729–738.

Lumley, M., Abeles, L., Melamed, B. G., Pistone, L., & Johnson, J. H. (1990). Coping outcomes in children facing stressful medical procedures: The role of child-environment variables. *Behavioral Assessment, 12,* 223–238.

Maddux, J. E., Roberts, M. C., Sledden, E. A., & Wright, L. (1986). Developmental issues in child health psychology. *American Psychologist, 41*(1), 25–34.

Melamed, B. G., Dearborn, M., & Hermecz, D. A. (1983). Necessary considerations for surgery preparation: Age and previous experience with the stressor. *Psychosomatic Medicine, 45,* 517–525.

Melamed, B. G., Meyer, R., Gee, C., & Soule, L. (1976). The influence of time and type of preparation on children's adjustment to hospitalization. *Journal of Pediatric Psychology,* 31–37.

Melamed, B. G., & Ridley-Johnson, R. (1988). Psychological preparation of families for hospitalization. *Journal of Developmental and Behavioral Pediatrics, 9,* 96–101.

Melamed, B. G., & Siegel, L. J. (1975). Reduction of anxiety in children facing hospitalization and surgery by use of filmed modeling. *Journal of Consulting and Clinical Psychology, 43*(4), 511–521.

Miller, S., Roussi, P., Caputo, G., & Kruns, L. (1995). Patterns of children's coping with an aversive dental treatment. *Health Psychology, 14*(3), 236–246.

Mischel, W., Shoda, Y., & Peake, P. K. (1988). The nature of adolescent competencies predicted by preschool delay of gratification. *Journal of Personality and Social Psychology, 54,* 687–696.

Moos, R. H. (Ed.). (1986). *Coping with life crises: An integrated approach.* New York: Plenum Press.

Olsen, K. H., McCubbin, H. I., Barnes, H., Larsen, A., Muzen, M., & Wilson, M. (1982). *Family inventories.* St Paul, MN: Family Social Science.

Olson, A., Johansen, S., Powers, L., Pope, J., & Klein, R. (1993). Cognitive coping strategies of children with chronic illness. *Developmental and Behavioral Pediatrics, 14,* 217–223.

Perrin, E. C., & Gerrity, S. (1981). There's a demon in your belly: Children's understanding of illness. *Pediatrics, 67*(6), 841–849.

Peterson, L., & Toler, S. M. (1986). An information seeking disposition in child surgery patients. *Health Psychology, 4,* 343–359.

Peterson, L. (1986). Coping by children undergoing stressful medical procedures: Some conceptual, methodological and therapeutic issues. *Journal of Consulting and Clinical Psychology, 57,* 380–387.

Rape, R. N., & Bush, J. P. (1994). Psychological preparations for pediatric oncology patients undergoing painful procedures: A methodological critique of the research. *Children's Health Care, 23*(1), 51–67.

Rehm, R. S. (2000). Parental encouragement, protection, and advocacy for Mexican-American children with chronic conditions. *Journal of Pediatric Nursing, 6,* 89–98.

Rodrigue, J., MacNaughton, B., Hoffman III, Graham-Pole, J., Andres, J., Novak, D., & Fennell, R. (1997). Transplantation in children: A longitudinal assessment of mother's stress. *Psychosomatics, 38,* 478–486.

Rosenstein, A. K., & Keefe, F. J. (1983). The use of coping strategies in chronic low back pain patients: Relationship to patient characteristics and current adjustment. *Pain, 17*(1), 33–44.

Ross, D. M., & Ross, S. A. (1988). Assessment of pediatric pain: An overview. *Issues in Comprehensive Pediatric Nursing, 11*(2–3), 73–91.

Rudolph, K. D., Denning, M. D., & Weisz, J. R. (1995). Determinants and consequences of children's coping in the medical setting: Conceptualization, review and critique. *Psychological Bulletin, 118,* 328–357.

Ryan-Wenger, N. M. (1992). A taxonomy of children's coping strategies: A step toward theory development. *American Journal of Orthopsychiatry, 62*(2), 257–263.

Seiffge-Krenke, I. (1998). Chronic disease and perceived developmental progression in adolescence. *Developmental Psychology, 34,* 1073–1084.

Sethi, A., Mischel, W., Aber, J. L., Shoda, Y., & Rodriguez, M. L. (2000). The role of strategic attention deployment in development of self-regulation: Predicting preschoolers' delay of gratification from mother-toddler interactions. *Developmental Psychology, 36*(6), 767–777.

Siegel, L., & Smith, K. (1991). Coping and adaptation of children's pain. In J. Bush & S. Hawkings (Eds.), *Children in pain: Clinical and research issues from a developmental perspective.* New York: Springer-Verlag.

Siegel, L. J., & Smith, K. E. (1989). Children's strategies for coping with pain. *Pediatrician, 16,* 110–118.

Spirito, A., Stark, L., Gil, K., & Tyc, V. (1995). Coping with everyday and disease-related stressors by chronically ill children and adolescents. *Journal of American Child and Adolescent Psychiatry, 34*(3), 283–290.

Spirito, A., Stark, L. J., & Williams, C. (1988). Development of a brief coping checklist for use with pediatric populations. *Journal of Pediatric Psychology, 13*(4), 555–574.

Suls, J., & Wan, C. K. (1989). Effects of sensory and procedural information on coping with stressful medical procedures and pain. A metanalysis. *Journal of Consulting and Clinical Psychology, 57,* 372–379.

Visintainer, M. A., & Wolfer, J. A. (1975). Psychological preparation for surgical pediatric patients: The effects on children's and parents' stress responses and adjustment. *Pediatrics, 56,* 187–202.

Weiss, K. L., Marvin, R. S., & Pianta, R. C. (1997). Ethnographic detection and description of family strategies for child care: Application to the study of cerebral palsy. *Journal of Pediatric Psychology, 22*(2), 263–278.

Wells, R. D., & Schwebel, A. I. (1987). Chronically ill children and their mothers: Predictors of resilience and vulnerability to hospitalization and surgical stress. *Developmental and Behavioral Pediatrics, 8,* 83–89.

Wertlieb, D., Weigel, C., & Feldstein, M. (1987). Measuring children's coping. *American Journal of Orthopsychiatry, 57*(4), 548–560.

Williams, P. D., Lorenzo, F. D., & Borja, M. (1993). Pediatric chronic illness: Effects on siblings and mothers. *Maternal Child Nursing Journal, 21*(4), 111–121.

Wolfer, J. A., & Visintainer, M. A. (1975). Pediatric surgical patients' and parents' stress responses and adjustment as a function of psychological preparation and stress-point nursing care. *Nursing Research, 24,* 244–255.

Wolfer, J. A., & Visintainer, M. A. (1979). Prehospital psychological preparation for tonsillectomy patients: Effects on children's and parent's adjustment. *Pediatrics, 64,* 646–655.

Wood, B. L. (1993). Beyond the "psychosomatic family": A biobehavioral family model of pediatric illness. *Family Process, 32*(3), 261–278.

Worchel, F., Copeland, D., & Barker, D. (1987). Control-related coping strategies in pediatric oncology patients. *Journal of Pediatric Psychology, 12*(1), 25–38.

CHAPTER 8

Adherence Research in the Pediatric and Adolescent Populations: A Decade in Review

Patricia V. Burkhart and Jacqueline Dunbar-Jacob

T he systematic study of adherence began in earnest in the 1970s. Since that time, researchers and clinicians have recognized the critical importance of adherence as it relates to health outcomes. Poor adherence to treatment continues to be a substantial problem affecting treatment outcomes and potentially increasing the likelihood of complications.

The objective of this chapter is to review the pediatric and adolescent adherence research during the last decade in order to evaluate the current status of the research and to examine trends over time. This review builds upon a previous examination from 1970–1989 of pediatric adherence research, to which the reader is referred for early research in the field (Dunbar-Jacob, Dunning, & Dwyer, 1993). For the purpose of this review, the words *adherence* and *compliance* are used interchangeably to mean the extent to which a person's behavior coincides with the proposed treatment regimen (Haynes, 1979). Articles were identified by authors and year of publication from 1987–1996. Corresponding to the previous review, information on age and size of sample, theoretical underpinnings, level of illness and disease, compliance behavior and measurement, and the study design are identified. The specific question posed for the systematic review of the literature is: What is the current state of knowledge in pediatric and adolescent adherence research? Trends in adherence research are discussed and related to current data from the National Center for Health Statistics (1994) and the objectives of Healthy People 2000 (1991).

METHOD OF REVIEW

Computer searches of Medline on-line and the Cumulative Index to Nursing and Allied Health Literature (CINAHL) were conducted using the key words patient adherence or compliance and child or adolescent. Attention was directed toward research articles focusing on compliance to treatment of an existing condition or a recommended prevention regimen. Studies on abstinence from substance abuse, alcohol, tobacco, or illicit drugs as well as compliance to birth control recommendations were not included. Review papers and comment or advice articles were excluded. Studies that included both adults and children in a combined analysis were also omitted. Relevant citations and abstracts were reviewed after which a total of 123 full text articles were screened. Sixty published research studies on pediatric and adolescent adherence, representing 58 separate investigations, were identified.

The articles are summarized by 5-year intervals. The findings were extracted by one reviewer and verified by the second reviewer. Characteristics of the pediatric adherence research studies were examined in relation to sample size, age of the sample, theoretical underpinnings, level of illness and disease, compliance behavior and measurement, compliance rate if reported, design type, whether the research used an experimental design, the intervention method if identified, the level of intervention, and improvement in compliance if reported for intervention studies.

CHARACTERISTICS OF THE STUDIES

Of the 60 published research papers related to pediatric or adolescent adherence (representing 58 separate investigations with different samples), 28 (representing 27 separate investigations) were published in the 5 years spanning 1987–1991 (see Table 8.1). Four to five studies were published during each of the 5 years except for the year 1990, when this number more than doubled to 11 published studies. Thirty-two articles, representing 31 different investigations were published during the 5-year interval from 1992–1996

TABLE 8.1 Pediatric Adherence Research Articles 1987–1991

Author	Year	Sample size	Age	Theory	Level of illness	Disease	Compliance behavior	Measure	Compliance rate	Design type	Exp	Intervention method	Level of intervention	Improvement
Anderson et al.	1990	121	6–21 yrs	—	Chronic	IDDM	CR	Self	—	C	No	—	—	—
Anson et al.	1990	43	4–19 yrs	—	Chronic	Celiac	Diet	Bio/ other	70% of patients	D	No	—	—	—
Birkhead et al.	1989	5	10–19 yrs	—	Chronic	Asthma	Meds	Bio	0% of patients	CS	No	—	—	—
Christiaanse et al.	1989	38	7–17 yrs	—	Chronic	Asthma	Meds	Bio	56% of patients	C	No	—	—	—
Cohen et al.	1991	26	1– > 15 yrs	Social sup/ stress	Chronic	Renal	Diet/meds	Bio	65.6% of patients	C	No	—	—	—
Creer et al.	1988	123	5–17 yrs	SLT	Chronic	Asthma	Meds/pefr	Self	57% M Comp	I	Yes	Ed/behavior (self-mgt./ model/tailor)	Parent/child	—
Delamater et al.	1988	33	$M = 14$ yrs	—	Chronic	IDDM	Diet	Self	42% of patients	D	No	—	—	—
Finney et al.	1990	8	4–17 yrs	—	Chronic	Allergy	Appt.	Chart	56% & 90% M Comp	I	No	Behavior (reward/ reminder)	Parent/child	+13%

(continued)

TABLE 8.1 *(continued)*

Author	Year	Sample size	Age	Theory	Level of illness	Disease	Compliance behavior	Measure	Compliance rate	Design type	Exp	Intervention method	Level of intervention	Improvement
Fraser	1990	155	Median 4.6 yrs	—	Prev	Varied	Immun.	Chart/self	72% & 85% of patients	D	No	—	—	—
Freund et al.	1991	68	6–19 yrs	—	Chronic	IDDM	CR	Self	Scale (5 Pt Sc)	D	No	—	—	—
Greenan-Fowler et al.	1987	10	8–15 yrs	—	Chronic	Hemophilia	Exercise	Self	55% M Comp	I	No	Ed/behavior (contracts rewards)	Parent/child	+39 Compliance
Hanna et al.	1990	55	6–18 yrs	Social action	Prev	CAD	Diet	Self/bio	—	D	No	—	—	—
Hanson et al.	1989	135	M 14.5 yrs	—	Chronic	IDDM	CR	Self/HCP	Scale (5 Pt Sc)	C	No	—	—	—
Hauser et al.	1990	52	M 12.8 yrs	—	Chronic	IDDM	CR	HCP/other	Scale (1–4 Sc)	D	No	—	—	—
Hazzard et al.	1990	35	9–16 yrs	—	Chronic	Epilepsy	Meds	Bio/other	44% of patients	C	No	—	—	—
Hudson et al.	1987	18	8–19 yrs	—	Chronic	Renal	CR	Self/other	Scale (1–4 Sc)	D	No	—	—	—
Hughes et al.	1991	89	6–16 yrs	—	Chronic	Asthma	Meds/PEFR	Self/bio	< 50% of patients	I	Yes	Ed/behavior (reinf/self-monitor)	Parent/child	—
Israel et al.	1987	54	8–13 yrs	—	Prev	Obesity	Weight	Self/mech	72% of patients	I	No	Ed/behavior (cues/rewards)	Parent/child	—

TABLE 8.1 *(continued)*

Author	Year	Sample size	Age	Theory	Level of illness	Disease	Compliance behavior	Measure	Compliance rate	Design type	Exp	Intervention method	Level of intervention	Improvement	Level of inter-vention
Jacobson et al.	1990	61	9–16 yrs	—	Chronic	IDDM	CR	HCP/other	Scale (4 Pt Sc)	D	No	—	—	—	—
Johnson et al.	1990	162	6–19 yrs	—	Chronic	IDDM	CR	Self	Scale (Hi/Lo)	C	No	—	—	—	—
Maiman et al.	1988	771	.5–10 yrs	—	Acute	Otitis	Meds	Self/pill ct	—	I	Yes	Physician Ed	MD	—	—
Marteau et al.	1987	65 Sets parent/child	5–16 yrs	HBM	Chronic	IDDM	CR	Other	—	C	No	—	—	—	—
Paynter et al.	1990	41	—	HBM	Chronic	Cleft palate	CR	Self	64.4% *M* Comp	D	No	—	—	—	—
Phipps & DeCuir-Whalley	1990	54	1 mo–20 yrs	—	Chronic	Varied	Meds	Chart	48% of patients	D	No	—	—	—	—
Pinzone et al.	1991	10	6–16 yrs	—	Chronic	Asthma	PEFR/meds	Self	—	C	No	—	—	—	—
Rapoff et al.	1988	3	3–13 yrs	—	Chronic	JRA	Meds	Self/pill ct	Scale (1–5 Sc)	CS	No	Ed/behavior (reinf/super-vision)	Parent	*M* +34% compliance	—
Taggart et al.	1987	12	4–12 yrs	SLT	Chronic	Asthma	Meds	Self	—	I	No	Ed/behavior (reinf/self-mgt)	Parent/child	—	—
Zora et al.	1989	17	5–13 yrs	—	Chronic	Asthma	Meds (in-haler)	Self/mech	8%–40% of patients	D	No	—	—	—	—

(continued)

TABLE 8.1 (*continued*)

Pediatric Adherence Research Articles Definition Guide

Theory	HBM = health belief model
	SLT = social learning theory
	Soc sup = social support
Level of illness	Prev = prevention
	Chronic = chronic illness
	Acute = acute illness
Disease	Ca = cancer
	CAD = coronary artery disease
	IDDM = insulin dependent diabetes mellitus
	Resp = respiratory
Compliance behavior	CR = complex regimen
	Meds = medications
	PEFR = peak expiratory flow rate
	Immuniz Rate = immunization rate

TABLE 8.1 (*continued*)

Measure of compliance behavior	Bio = biological assay
	Elec = electronic
	HCP = health care provider
	Mech = mechanical
	Pill Ct = pill count
	Self = self-report
Compliance rate	M Comp = mean compliance
Design	C = correlation
	CS = case study
	D = descriptive
	I = intervention
Exp	No = experimental design
	Yes = non-experimental design
Intervention method	Behav = behavior
	Ed = education
	Mod = modification
Level of intervention	Par = parent

(see Table 8.2). There appears to be a leveling off in the number of pediatric adherence studies, with 10 publications in the years 1992 and 1993, and 6 papers published in 1994. In the years 1995 and 1996, only three studies appeared in the literature. Just why the interest or attention to adherence among the young has stabilized at such a low rate is not clear, particularly in light of newer measurement technology and the paucity of intervention research (see Tables 8.1 and 8.2).

Sample Sizes and Age Levels

Sample size was listed for each study. Sample sizes have increased over time. During the period from 1987–1991, the 27 studies had sample sizes ranging from 3–771. The median sample size was 43. Approximately half (52%, n = 14) had sample sizes > 50. For the interval 1992–1996, the 31 published studies identified sample sizes ranging from 8–1997. The median sample size was 75. The majority (61%, n = 19) of the studies stated sample sizes > 50 subjects.

Throughout the decade, most of the studies addressed the age groups of school-age through adolescence. Few (19%, n = 5) articles focused on infants or toddlers unless they were included with all pediatric age groups in the study. During 1987–1991 the school-age and adolescent populations were addressed jointly in 22 (81%) of the 27 studies. Similarly, during the second half of the decade, 1992–1996, the proportion of research focused on school-age and adolescent children far outweighed those sampling infants and toddlers. In contrast to the early part of the decade, there was a shift toward more interest focused on the adolescent population. Seven (23%) of the 29 studies sampled adolescents alone, while 15 (48%) identified school-age children and adolescents together. Two (6%) of the articles focused only on school-age children to study compliance behavior. In the 1970s, more young children were studied since the focus of the compliance strategies was the parent. An important shift took place in the 1980s when self-management programs began to evolve. Children's adherence behaviors, rather than those of their parents, became the focus of study. Therefore, the shift to research of the older child may parallel the trend in program development.

Use of Theory

The majority of the pediatric adherence research is atheoretical. This pattern has not changed over time. During the past decade, 13 (22%) of the 58

TABLE 8.2 Pediatric Adherence Research Articles (1992–1996)

Author	Year	Sample size	Age	Theory	Level of illness	Disease	Compliance behavior	Compliance Measure	Compliance rate	Design type	Exp	Intervention method	Level of intervention	Improvement
Alessandro et al.	1994	257	2–15 yrs	—	Chronic	Asthma	Meds	Self	63% of patients	D	No	—	—	—
Bartsch et al.	1993	77	9–14 yrs	—	Acute	Ortho-dontic	Appliance	Elec	57% M Comp	C	No	—	—	—
Boardway et al.	1993	19	12–17 yrs	—	Chronic	IDDM	CR	Self/bio	Scale	I	Yes	Ed/behavior (Stress Mgt.)	Parent/child	—
Bond et al.	1992	56	10–19 yrs	HBM	Chronic	IDDM	CR	Self	Scale (1–5 Sc)	C	No	—	—	—
Brown-bridge & Fielding	1994	60	2–21 yrs	—	Chronic	Renal	CR	Self/bio/other	Scale (0 = hi/ 0–35 sc)	C	No	—	—	—
Burkhart	1996	42	7–11 yrs	SLT	Chronic	Asthma	PEFR	Elec/self	58.5% M Comp	I	Yes	Ed/behavior (contract/re-inf/rewards/cues)	Parent/child	+11.4% comp
Burroughs et al.	1993	21	13–18 yrs	—	Chronic	IDDM	CR	Self	Scale (1–4 Sc)	C	No	—	—	—
Charron-Prochownik et al.	1993	50	6–9 yrs	HBM	Chronic	IDDM	CR	Self/bio/other	Scale	C	No	—	—	—
Coutts et al.	1992	14	9–16 yrs	—	Chronic	Asthma	Meds (Inhaled)	Self/elec	43% M Comp	D	No	—	—	—

(continued)

TABLE 8.2 *(continued)*

Author	Year	Sample size	Age	Theory	Level of illness	Disease	Compliance behavior	Compliance Measure	Compliance rate	Design type	Exp	Intervention method	Level of intervention	Improvement
D'Angelo et al.	1992	29	8–18 yrs	—	Chronic	Hemo-philia	CR	Self/HCP	Scale	C	No	—	—	—
Daviss et al.	1995	79	10–16 yrs	—	Chronic	IDDM	Diet	Self	Scale (1–5 Sc)	C	No	—	—	—
Drozda et al.	1993	179	4–23 yrs	—	Chronic	IDDM	Urine Collection	Bio	—	I	Yes	Ed/behavior (reminder/phone)	Parent/child	+
Engel	1993	8	9–15 yrs	—	Chronic	Head-ache	Relaxation/Meds	Self/pill ct	84% & 100% M Comp	CS	No	—	—	—
Festa et al.	1992	50	12.9–25.6 yrs	—	Chronic	Ca	Meds	Bio	50% & 52% of patients	D	No	—	—	—
Foulkes et al.	1993	32	6–21 yrs	—	Chronic	Renal	Meds	Bio/pill ct	—	C	No	—	—	—
Hanson et al.	1992	95	11–22 yrs	SLT Family Systems	Chronic	IDDM	Diet	Self	—	C	No	—	—	—
Hentinen & Kyngas	1992	47	15–17 yrs	—	Chronic	IDDM	CR	Self/bio	34% of patients	D	No	—	—	—
Johnson & Kelly	1992	193	M = 11.9 yrs	—	Chronic	IDDM	CR	Self	—	C	No	—	—	—

TABLE 8.2 (*continued*)

Author	Year	Sample size	Age	Theory	Level of illness	Disease	Compliance behavior	Measure	Compliance rate	Design type	Exp	Intervention method	Level of intervention	Improvement
Kovacs et al.	1992	95	8–21 yrs	—	Chronic	IDDM	CR	Self/ HCP	70.5% of patients	D	No	—	—	—
Kovacs et al.	1995	92	8–21 yrs	—	Chronic	IDDM	CR	Self/ HCP	61% of patients	C	No	—	—	—
LaGreca et al.	1995	74	11–18 yrs	—	Chronic	IDDM	CR	Self	Scale (0–41 Sc)	D	No	—	—	—
Loprei- ato & Ot- tolini	1996	1977	2–18 yrs	—	Prev	—	Immuniz. rate	Chart	84% of patients	D	No	—	—	—
Manne et al.	1993	77	3–10 yrs	—	Chronic	CR	CR	HCP	51.9% appt. keeping of patients	C	No	—	—	—
Miller- Johnson et al.	1994	88	8–18 yrs	—	Chronic	IDDM	CR	Self/ HCP	Scale (0–100 Sc)	C	No	—	—	—
Paynter et al.	1993	30	7 mo– 16 yrs	HBM	Chronic	Cleft palate	CR	Self	82% M comp (56.7% of patients)	D	No	—	—	—

(*continued*)

TABLE 8.2 *(continued)*

Author	Year	Sample size	Age	Theory	Level of illness	Disease	Compliance behavior	Measure	Compliance rate	Design type	Exp	Intervention method	Level of intervention	Improvement
Reid et al.	1994	56	8–18 yrs	Approach/coping	Chronic	IDDM	Diet/glucose	Self	Scale (0–5 Sc)	C	No	—	—	—
Schlundt et al.	1994	20	13–19 yrs	—	Chronic	IDDM	Diet	Self	—	D	No	—	—	—
Schoni et al.	1995	89	2 mo–14 yrs	—	Acute/chronic	Resp	Meds	Bio/elec	47% M Comp	D	No	—	—	—
Szilagyi et al.	1992	124	1–18 yrs	HBM/LOC	Prev	Asthma	Vaccination	Chart	7% of patients	I	Yes	Behav/(reminder)	Parent	+23% compliance
Tamaroff et al.	1992	34	12.9–25.6 yrs	—	Chronic	Ca	Meds	Self/bio	50% of patients	D	No	—	—	—
Wysocki et al.	1992	81	18–22 yrs	—	Chronic	IDDM	CR	Self	Score on 15 item test	C	No	—	—	—
Wysocki et al.	1996	100	5–17 yrs	—	Chronic	IDDM	CR	Self	Score on test	C	No	—	—	—

TABLE 8.2 *(continued)*

Pediatric Adherence Research Articles Definition Guide

Theory	HBM = health belief model
	SLT = social learning theory
	Soc sup = social support
Level of illness	Prev = prevention
	Chronic = chronic illness
	Acute = acute illness
Disease	Ca = cancer
	CAD = coronary artery disease
	IDDM = insulin dependent diabetes mellitus
	Resp = respiratory
Compliance behavior	CR = complex regimen
	Meds = medications
	PEFR = peak expiratory flow rate
	Immuniz Rate = immunization rate

(continued)

TABLE 8.2 *(continued)*

Measure of compliance behavior	Bio = biological assay
	Elec = electronic
	HCP = health care provider
	Mech = mechanical
	Pill Ct = pill count
	Self = self-report
Compliance rate	*M* Comp = mean compliance
Design	C = correlation
	CS = case study
	D = descriptive
	I = intervention
Exp	No = experimental design
	Yes = non-experimental design
Intervention method	Behav = behavior
	Ed = education
	Mod = modification
Level of intervention	Par = parent

investigations were theory driven. Dunbar-Jacob, Dunning, and Dwyer (1993) found 21% of studies published from 1970–1989 identified theoretical under-pinnings. Of the current studies guided by theoretical formulations, the Health Belief Model (46%, n = 6) continues to predominate, followed by Social Learning Theory (30%, n = 4). Health locus of control, approach-coping, family systems, stress-coping, and social support theories have also made an appearance in the pediatric adherence literature in isolated studies.

There is a critical need to use theory and to test it systematically so that pieces of information on pediatric adherence form a comprehensive knowledge base. Additionally, it is important to recognize that theoretical constructs and principles that describe adult behavior may not be adequate to describe the behavior of children. Indeed, the use of developmental frame-works may also be useful in setting the stage for the capabilities of the child or parent to manage treatment regimen. Theories are beneficial as a basis for predicting or explaining children's adherence behaviors.

Illness Focus

Children with chronic conditions continue to be the major focus of pediatric adherence studies in 50 (86%) of the 58 articles. Adherence to preventive therapy was identified in only 5 (9%) of the studies. Acute illness has generated little interest with only 2 (3%) of the studies measuring compliance to acute illness treatment alone and a third study (Schoni, Horak, & Nikolaizik, 1995) evaluating compliance to treatment in both acute and chronic respiratory conditions. The focus on chronic conditions is a shift from that of the early 1970s, during which time two thirds of the pediatric compliance research was directed toward acute illness (Dunbar et al., 1993). This trend continued from the late 1970s into the 1990s.

Within chronic conditions, researchers spotlighted diabetes and asthma. During the first half of the decade, 7 (26%) of the studies addressed diabetes and the same number dealt with asthma. By the second half of the decade, the number of studies in which the focus was diabetes treatment compliance totaled 17 (55%), whereas only 4 (13%) focused on asthma. The disparity between diabetes and asthma research is a striking contrast considering asthma is the most prevalent chronic condition affecting children. An estimated 7% of children in the United States under the age of 18 have asthma, whereas < 1% of children under 18 years are diagnosed with diabetes (National Center for Health Statistics, 1994). Furthermore, there continues to be an alarming increase in asthma morbidity and mortality rates (Weiss, Gergen, & Hodgson,

1992); 4.8 million children in the U.S. are affected by the disease (National Center for Health Statistics, 1995).

Other chronic illnesses such as renal conditions, celiac disease, hemophilia, obesity, allergy, chronic bronchitis, headache, cancer, epilepsy, and cleft palate were addressed predominantly in single studies. Pediatric compliance research would benefit from the study of a range of chronic conditions in children, particularly, those conditions occurring with increased frequency. Treatment regimens vary across conditions, and it is not clear whether contributions to poor adherence or strategies to improve adherence generalize across not only the age ranges affected but also the common chronic conditions of childhood. As previously mentioned, asthma is the most prevalent pediatric chronic condition, affecting 7% of children. Asthma is followed by sinusitis and allergic conditions (6.5% and 6%, respectively), dermatitis and acne (3.8% and 2.9%, respectively), and orthopedic impairments (2.8%). Other chronic diseases of children are those affecting the tonsils or adenoids, speech impairment, heart disease, and hearing defects (National Center for Health Statistics, 1994).

The two acute illness studies focused on otitis media and orthodontics, reflecting a paucity of adherence research in the area of acute illness. According to the National Center for Health Statistics (1994), the acute illness incidence rates per 100 persons per year in children under the age of 5 years rank as follows: respiratory conditions (153.8), acute ear infections (62.7), infective and parasitic diseases (54.7), injuries (25.4), and digestive system conditions (10.5). In children ages 5–17, respiratory conditions (103.4) predominate followed by infective and parasitic diseases (41.9), injuries (26.0), acute ear infections (13.66), and digestive system conditions (8.3).

The 5 prevention studies considered immunization or vaccination rates as well as dietary prevention of obesity and coronary heart disease in single studies. Studies devoted to the important aspect of prevention have been largely neglected. Considering the importance given to prevention of illness and disease identified by Healthy People 2000: National Health Promotion and Disease Prevention Objectives (U.S. Department of Health & Human Services, 1991), more research on the utilization of clinical preventive practices is needed.

Adherence Behaviors Addressed

In the first half of the decade, medication adherence was the focus of compliance behaviors studied in 37% (n = 10) of the research articles. Adherence to complex regimens was identified in 30% (n = 8) of the studies. Dietary adherence (15%, n = 3) ranked third. The second half of the decade saw a shift to the study of complex or multicomponent regimens in the majority (52%, n = 16) of the studies, paralleling the influx of diabetes research. Glucose monitoring, diet, exercise, and insulin administration were included among the complex behaviors of the diabetes articles. Complex regimens related to the four specific conditions of hemophilia, cancer, renal disease, and cleft palate were addressed in single studies. Medications (n = 6, 19% of studies) and diet (n = 4, 13% of studies) followed second and third as compliance behaviors of interest in the second half of the decade. Of lesser importance to researchers throughout the decade were appointment keeping, self-monitoring (e.g., peak expiratory flow rate in two studies, glucose testing, and urine collecting), appliance wearing, immunization rates in 3 studies, and relaxation. Similar to the findings of the 1970s and 1980s (Dunbar et al., 1993), the 1990s addressed few compliance behaviors in very few illnesses.

Measurement of Adherence

Self-report continues to play a significant role as a measure of adherence behaviors. Of the 58 separate investigations, 36% (n = 21) relied on self-report alone as the compliance assessment strategy. Little change from this pattern was evident when comparing the first to the second half of the decade. In fact, compliance measures overall were consistent throughout the decade. Self-report was also used in combination with other objective measures in several studies. Although self-report has been noted to have a bias toward overestimation among adults, the accuracy of self-report in pediatric populations has not been systematically examined.

In some studies, self-report was followed by biological assays (24%, n = 14) as a measure of adherence. Health care provider (HCP) observations were employed as a measure of adherence in 12% (n = 7) of the articles. To a lesser extent, pill counts (7%, n = 4), chart reviews (7%, n = 4), and mechanical measures (e.g., weight of canister or scale) were used. Several of the studies utilized more than one measure of compliance. Although it was predicted that the 1990s would see an increase in electronically measured compliance, this was not the case. Only 4 (7%) of the studies utilized computerized equipment to measure adherence objectively. Considering the problems inherent in self-reporting, including the issue of accuracy, it is surprising that this method continues to predominate.

During the decade spanning 1987–1996, surprisingly, just 83% (n = 48) of the 58 published studies reported compliance rates. The 10 studies not reporting adherence rates identified factors associated with or predicting adherence rather than the actual adherence data. Of the 48 studies that did report adherence rates, 19% (n = 9) identified the mean adherence rate, that is, the average percentage of the regimen actually carried out by subjects. Forty-two percent (n = 20) of the papers presented the adherence rate as the percentage of patients who complied with treatment based on predetermined criteria for adherence, while the remaining 37% (n = 18) identified the rate based on a predetermined scale.

Upon examination of pediatric compliance research, a salient feature is the inconsistency in reporting compliance rates. In addition to the 10 studies not reporting patient compliance rates, others determined compliance qualitatively, based on an investigator-generated scale developed specifically for that study, or stated a percentage of compliant patients based on a cutoff point for good compliance. This trend is problematic, making comparative assessments of adherence across conditions difficult, if not impossible. "Probably the most informative definition [of compliance] is the percentage of the regimen actually carried out. This allows the reader to draw his own conclusions regarding acceptable levels of compliance" (Dunbar, 1983, p. 211).

When reported mean adherence rates were calculated, they ranged from 43%–100%. The median was 58%. The range for the percentage of patients adhering to recommended treatment was from 0%–85% of patients. The median number of patients adhering to prescribed regimen was 51%. Although the range of average adherence rates for this decade was higher than in previous decades (Dunbar-Jacob et al., 1993), the median adherence rate was consistent with the 1970s and 1980s, persisting at around 55%.

Study Designs for Pediatric Adherence

Of the 58 research studies reviewed, correlational (41%, n = 24) and descriptive (35%, n = 20) design types predominated. Only 19% (n = 11) were intervention studies. Five percent (n = 3) of the articles were case studies. Seven (64%) of the intervention studies used an experimental design, including adequate control conditions, randomization, and manipulation of the independent variable.

The number of intervention studies represented a decline in this design type from the previous 2 decades (Dunbar-Jacob et al., 1993). The decade showed correlational studies gaining in popularity as compared with the 1970s and 1980s. Most of the correlational studies focused on specific behaviors, psychosocial, or demographic variables as determinants of health behavior compliance.

It appears there is still much to learn about specific interventions that would improve compliance. The lack of intervention studies may be due to a publication bias, in that positive findings related to specific intervention strategies are likely to appear in the published literature, whereas negative findings are less likely to be published.

Intervention Methods Employed

The type of interventions has remained consistent for different time periods. Multicomponent interventions grew in favor in the 1980s and continue today. Educational and behavioral strategies were represented in 72% (n = 8) of the intervention studies, and in one case study. The majority of the behavioral interventions were multicomponent strategies. Single behavioral strategies (18%, n = 2) were scarce. In only one study was education used alone to improve physicians' adherence-related knowledge and behavior. Compliance rates improved an average of 25% in the 6 studies reporting improvement rates when behavioral strategies were employed.

A major gap exists in the type of methodologies employed in adherence research. There is a paucity of intervention studies, in particular, those using rigorous experimental designs to examine the relative contribution of various behavioral strategies to the enhancement of pediatric compliance. The lack of attention to this endeavor has made it difficult to generalize successful outcomes to the practice setting.

The target population for intervention in pediatric adherence continues to be the parent and child in 75% of the study designs employing an intervention strategy. To a lesser degree, parents (17%, n = 2) and the physicians (8%, n = 1) were addressed as the focus of the interventions. A focus on the parent and child dyad reflects the growing body of knowledge indicating the importance of parent involvement in the child's adherence.

DEVELOPMENTAL ISSUES RELATED TO ADHERENCE

Research directed toward understanding adherence in the pediatric and adolescent populations must take developmental issues into account. Age-specific differences influence children's ability to comprehend, acquire, and perform skills necessary for management of health-related activities.

Infant and toddler adherence to advised treatment regimens is largely determined by the ability of the parent or guardian to understand and follow through with health care provider recommendations. As age increases, children have the cognitive capability to carry out treatment tasks. According to Piaget (1951), school-age children (7–12 years) are moving from sensory-motor to conceptual learning. The emphasis on cognitive competencies allows children to comprehend and symbolize critical elements in their lives. Children begin to think and reason about events and objects, memory increases, and language competence becomes more extensive. School-age children engage in the developmental task of industry (Erikson, 1963), learning to regulate their own behavior, and to some extent, control the environment rather than being controlled by it. As children enter school, they begin to move away from their parents and home environment. Peers and outside activities shift to the forefront.

As children enter and progress through adolescence, they achieve greater autonomy, seeking independence and challenging the authority of their parents. A developing capacity for formal abstract operations (Piaget, 1951) provides the foundation for individuation and separation from the family. Concurrently, adolescents struggle with self-esteem, body image, social role definition, and peer-related issues.

The increasing numbers of single-parents and working parents along with the shift in health care toward consumer self-management for disease prevention and health promotion, has created a situation of placing increasing responsibility on the school-age child and adolescent. Assigning too much responsibility for treatment management on the child may lead to noncompliance.

The literature reported in Tables 8.1 and 8.2 was examined for age-related differences in adherence. Adolescents were typically less adherent than their younger counterparts. Adherence to treatment regimen was found to deteriorate with increasing age (i.e., adolescence) in children with diabetes (Anderson, Auslander, Jung, Miller, & Santiago, 1990; Jacobson et al., 1990; Bond, Aiken, & Somerville, 1992; Drozda, Allen, Turner, Slusher, & McCain, 1993; Hanson, De Guire, Schinkel, & Henngeler, 1992; Johnson et al., 1992; Reid, Dubow, Carey, & Dura, 1994) and children with asthma (Christiaanse, Lavigne, & Lerner, 1989). Similarly, in a longitudinal study (n = 52), preadolescents (9–12 years) were found to be more adherent to the diabetic regimen at study entry than adolescents (13–16 years) (Jacobson et al., 1990). Adolescents tended to show poorer adherence than younger children (p < .001) in a sample of 60 children in end-stage renal failure undergoing dialysis (Brownbridge & Fielding, 1994). Average age of first onset of noncompliance was found to be 14.8 years (range 11.0–17.9 years) in a study of 95 children with insulin-dependent diabetes mellitus, with 17–19 year-olds being associated with the most amount of time being nonadherent (Kovacs, Goldston, Obrosky, & Iyengar, 1992).

Conversely, Phipps and DeCuir-Whalley (1990) found greater nonadherence to oral antibiotic regimen following bone marrow transplantation for cancer treatment in preschool and school-age children (n = 54) than in adolescents. This was consistent with the findings of a sample (n = 32) of children receiving immunosuppressant therapy for renal transplantation. Compared with older children, younger children were found to be less compliant (p < .005) with the multiple drug regimen (Foulkes, Boggs, Fennell, & Skibinski, 1993).

Although the findings for the relationship between age and adherence remain equivocal, developmental issues do generally appear to play a significant role in a child's willingness and ability to comply with medical advice. As children get older, they gradually become less dependent upon their parents and are expected to assume greater control over all aspects of their lives. Adolescents may exercise noncompliance in an attempt to test the limits and restrictions resulting from their disease, as a response to peer pressure, denial, or based on perceived changes in body image related to treatment. Age-related barriers to treatment compliance as well as specific personal and family characteristics that support adherence need to be explored. Research focused on the important role of parental mentoring, supervision, and guidance as it relates to the phenomenon of child and adolescent compliance is needed.

In a recent study of the adherence of school-age children with asthma, children were asked what helped them to remember to comply with self-monitoring, using a peak flow meter, on a daily basis. Twenty-seven (64%) of the children (n = 42) responded that parents' reminders helped them to remember to perform the requisite behavior (Burkhart, 1996). In the same study, accuracy in the self-reporting of data in a diary, based on the child's electronically recorded peak flow rate value, declined over time. Children sometimes wrote higher or lower numbers or made up values to write in their diaries that were not electronically recorded. These events occurred despite the researcher's admonition to parents to supervise the children's performances of the behaviors. As time went on, parents tended to rely solely on the children to perform the behavior appropriately. This resulted in inaccurate self-reporting and noncompliance.

These findings underscore the value of parental supervision for children in the performance of health behaviors. Shared family responsibility for treatment regimens appears to be an important element for consistent adherence to treatment in the pediatric population (Anderson, Auslander, Jung, Miller, & Santiago, 1990).

FACTORS AFFECTING ADHERENCE

Determinants of adherence have continued to interest researchers. Although many factors may be associated with low adherence, none has consistently been shown to be a significant predictor of compliance. The age variable has already been discussed in the previous section on developmental issues related to adherence. Most of the findings from the studies that explored an association between various demographic and psychosocial factors and adherence were correlational and inconclusive. Gender was not found to be correlated with adherence (Bartsch, Witt, Sahm, & Schneider, 1993; Hazzard, Hutchinson, & Krawiecki, 1990; Hentinen & Kyngas, 1992; Phipps & DeCuir-Whalley, 1990; Kovacs, Charron-Prochownik, & Obrosky, 1995; Miller-Johnson, Emery, Marvin, Clarke, Lovinger, & Martin, 1994; and Tamaroff, Festa, Adesman, & Walco, 1992). In several studies, greater adherence was associated with higher socioeconomic status (Charron-Prochownik, Becker, Brown, Liang, & Bennett, 1993; Manne, Jacobsen, Gorfinkle, Gerstein, & Redd, 1993; and Miller-Johnson et al., 1994). Conversely, others found no statistically significant relationship between adherence and socioeconomic status (Kovacs, Goldston, Obrosky, & Iyengar, 1992, and Wysocki et al., 1996).

Various family factors have also been explored. In a study of children (n = 60) undergoing dialysis for renal disease (Brownbridge & Fielding, 1994), low treatment adherence was associated with family structure (p < .01). That is, children not living with both natural parents tended to be less compliant. High levels of general family flexibility predicted positive dietary adherence in diabetic children (Hanson et al., 1992) and a supportive parenting style resulted in fewer adherence problems for children undergoing cancer treatment (Manne et al., 1993). In a 4-year longitudinal study of children with diabetes (n = 52) aged 9–16 years, children's and parents' perceptions of family conflict were strongly associated with low adherence, levels whereas perceived family cohesion predicted higher levels of adherence (Hauser, Jacobson, Lavori, Wolfsdorf, Herskowitz, Milley, & Bliss, 1990). An increased report of family conflict was also associated with nonadherence to diabetic regimen in a study of children (n = 88) aged 8–18 years (Miller-Johnson et al., 1994). Similarly, although no relationship was found between social support of the parent and the child's compliance with medication, a significant positive relationship was found between the number of stressful life events and noncompliance to medications for renal transplant recipients (n = 32) (Foulkes, Boggs, Fennell, & Skibinski, 1993). Additionally, parental anxiety was associated with lower rates of medication compliance for children with seizure disorders (Hazzard, Hutchinson, & Krawiecki, 1990). The findings on demographic and social variables have been inconsistent. However, they signaled the possibility that under certain treatment conditions, any of the sociodemographic variables may be implicated in nonadherence.

Psychosocial variables that may affect a child's adherence have also been examined. Two constructs that have received some attention in the research on children's adherence are locus of control and self-concept. *Locus of control* refers to the perception that an outcome will be largely determined by the individual's own actions (internal locus of control) or dependent on external forces (external locus of control) beyond the individual's control (Rotter, 1954). *Self-concept* (i.e., self-esteem) is a composite view of oneself (Bandura, 1986). Neither locus of control nor self-concept were consistently found to be associated with adherence in the studies reviewed. Szilagyi, Rodewald, Savageau, Yoos, and Doane (1992) analyzed the differences in health locus of control scores before and after an intervention to enhance compliance to immunizations in children with asthma. The authors found no significant change in locus of control. No statistically significant difference was found by means of an independent t-test when compliers and noncompliers to medication were compared, based on their health locus of control in a sample of adolescents with cancer (Tamaroff, Festa, Adesman, & Walco, 1992). Similarly, no association was found between health locus of control and the prediction of adherence to peak flow monitoring in school-age children with asthma (Burkhart, 1996). In contrast, a small pediatric asthma self-management study (n = 12) demonstrated a significant change in health locus of control toward internality for school-age children participating in the program (Taggart, Zuckerman, Lucas, Acty-Lindsey, & Bellanti, 1987).

The condition itself may be a factor in determining whether internal or external locus of control influences adherence. Bartch, Witt, Sahm, and Schneider (1993) studied a sample (n = 77) of children aged 9–14 years for patient compliance in wearing removable appliances for orthodontal problems. Parental external locus of control was found to be closely related to adherence. In a study of children with diabetes, the authors reported that those who had a greater internal locus of control exhibited greater adherence to treatment (Jacobson et al., 1990). These studies raise provocative questions regarding the association between locus of control and adherence, laying the foundation for future research.

The research conducted on the relationship between self-concept and adherence has also been inconclusive. Cognitive social learning theory posits that self-concept contributes to the individual's cognitive appraisal of his or her ability to perform specific behaviors (Bandura, 1986). Ferrand and Cox (1993) used regression analysis to assess the contributions of specific sociodemographic variables to health behaviors of preadolescent children (n = 260). Health perception was the single consistent variable affecting health behavior, and self-concept directly affected health perception. As part of a randomized, controlled intervention study for adherence to peak flow monitoring in school-age children (n = 42) with asthma, Burkhart (1996) examined self-concept as a moderating factor in the prediction of adherence to peak flow monitoring. Self-concept, measured by the Piers-Harris Children's Self-Concept Scale (Piers & Harris, 1984), was found to contribute to predicting subsequent adherence to electronic peak flow monitoring. Burkhart advises, however, that the results should be interpreted with caution, since the less conservative p value (p < .05) was used with multiple comparisons generating spearman correlation coefficients. Of particular interest were the anxiety subscale (r_s = .38, p = .014) and the intellectual and school status subscale (r_s = .38, p = .012) that were found to be positively related to daily adherence to peak flow monitoring. High scores on these subscales suggested perceived achievement, capability, and low anxiety may be associated with adherence. Perhaps these scores reflect the concept identified by Bandura (1977) as self-efficacy, the perception that one can successfully execute behavior required to produce a desired outcome. Greater adherence was found to be associated with higher child self-efficacy in a sample (n = 50) of school-age children with diabetes (Charron-Prochownik et al., 1993).

The psychosocial variables have been measured predominantly using correlational statistics or regression analyses from which causal relationships with adherence cannot be inferred. Research is needed in this area employing controlled, experimental study designs and standardized instruments with robust reliability and validity. Children's health locus of control and self-concept, including self-efficacy, may have clinical significance if in future studies they are found to affect children's adherence to treatment. Given the inconsistencies found and the paucity of studies examining such constructs as locus of control, self-concept, health belief, and self-efficacy in relation to adherence, future research in this area is warranted.

SUMMARY AND IMPLICATIONS FOR CLINICAL PRACTICE AND FUTURE RESEARCH

The promise of expanding research to further our understanding of pediatric adherence has only partially been met. While a steady rate of studies has been reported over the past decade, the rise in measurement technology and the need for scientifically-based interventions has not promoted the level of attention that the rates of nonadherence call for. Just 52% of children, on average, adhere to treatment. These rates hold for children with serious disorders such as cancer, chronic conditions with potential long-term adverse consequences such as asthma and diabetes, prevention practices such as immunization, as well as such acute and less serious disorders as respiratory infections.

Interestingly, the research over the past decade continues to rely heavily upon self-report methods of adherence. In the adult populations, this method has been shown to overestimate adherence. Among the pediatric populations these methods may be even more suspect, given the reliance on children who may not have the cognitive capability to adequately self-monitor or the parent who may or may not be intimately involved with event by event aspects of the treatment regimen. With the advent and increasing use of electronic event monitoring for varying aspects of a treatment regimen in the adult population, increasing attention to this technology is called for in pediatrics. Along with this is the need for an examination of the utility of self-report measures in this population.

There is an additional need for consistency in the reporting of adherence behaviors. Nineteen percent of the studies addressing compliance failed to report compliance rates at all. For the remaining studies, a variety of methods were used to classify patients as adherent. This continues to make comparisons across studies difficult and to limit the amount of knowledge attained about compliance.

Further limiting the knowledge gained about compliance in pediatrics is the limited attention to relevant theory guiding the studies. The research over this decade has suffered from lack of attention to theoretically based investigation, particularly the utilization of developmentally-based theory to guide the research on predictors as well as on interventions. The work that has been done shows little differentiation from the research on adults in terms of the selection of theory and the identification of predictors of adherence. Yet we know that children are not small adults. Their cognitive capabilities, ability to self-manage and to conceptualize the future consequences of their behavior, as well as to self-monitor, vary considerably over the range from infancy through adolescence. Additionally, more than their adult counterparts, the child and adolescent are following treatment regimens within the context of a family environment and often with considerable if not complete family involvement. Family functioning theories may be of particular interest in examining the adherence of the child. Indeed, what research exists suggests that developmental and family influences on adherence among children is of considerable importance.

A particular disappointment over the past decade is the limited attention to intervention research. Where behavioral intervention has been studied improvement rates have been substantial. Yet the proportion of research devoted to remediating this significant problem in health care has been minimal. There is a need to identify developmentally appropriate interventions for various family configurations if health care is to be improved for children.

Although progress has been made in understanding and modifying adherence among pediatric populations, there remains much to be learned. Progress in this area will be dependent upon the involvement of the interdisciplinary team in managing care as well as designing research. At the core is the physician responsible for planning, with the family, the care to be undertaken. Other health team members will vary dependent upon the conditions and the specific regimens of interest, for example, the nurse providing discharge instruction, patient education and/or home care, the dietitian, the physical therapist, the exercise physiologist, or other health care providers. Of particular relevance to the pediatric group would be professional expertise in child development, family functioning, behavioral interventions, and educational strategies with children and adolescents. As interdisciplinary expertise is brought to bear on the research issues related to the problem of adherence in pediatrics, we would expect to see the gaps in our understanding begin to close.

Over time there has been an increased emphasis on chronic disorders and on the older child using self-management strategies, yet a number of conditions and regimen behaviors are underrepresented in the literature. There remains a need for improved measurement technologies as well as for the use of developmental and family theories in the identification of predictors and intervention techniques. Overall there remains a glaring need for the development of scientifically-based interventions for varying developmental levels and for varying family configurations.

REFERENCES

Alessandro, F., Vincenzo, Z., Marco, S., Marcello, G., & Enrica, R. (1994). Compliance with pharmacologic prophylaxis and therapy in bronchial asthma. *Annals of Allergy, 73*(2), 135–140.

Anderson, B., Auslander, W., Jung, K., Miller, J., & Santiago, J. (1990). *Journal of Pediatric Psychology, 15*(4), 477–492.

Anson, O., Weizman, Z., & Zeevi, N. (1990). Celiac disease: Parental knowledge and attitudes of dietary compliance. *Pediatrics, 85*(1), 98–103.

Bandura, A. (1977). Self-efficacy: Toward a unifying theory of behavior change. *Psychological Review, 84*, 191–215.

Bandura, A. (1986). *Social foundations of thought and action: A social cognitive theory.* Englewood Cliffs, NJ: Prentice-Hall.

Bartsch, A., Witt, E., Sahm, G., & Schneider, S. (1993). Correlates of objective patient compliance with removable appliance wear. *American Journal of Orthodontics and Dentofacial Orthopedics, 104*(4), 378–386.

Birkhead, G., Attaway, N., Strunk, R., Townsend, M., & Teutsch, S. (1989). Investigation of a cluster of deaths of adolescents from asthma: Evidence implicating inadequate treatment and poor patient adherence with medications. *Journal of Allergy and Clinical Immunology, 84*(4), 484–491.

Boardway, R., Delamater, A., Tomakowsky, J., & Gutai, J. (1993). Stress management training for adolescents with diabetes. *Journal of Pediatric Psychology, 18*(1), 29–45.

Bond, G., Aiken, L., & Somerville, S. (1992). The health belief model and adolescents with insulin-dependent diabetes mellitus. *Health Psychology, 11*(3), 190–198.

Brownbridge, G., & Fielding, D. (1994). Psychosocial adjustment and adherence to dialysis treatment regimes. *Pediatric Nephrology, 8*, 744–749.

Burkhart, P. (1996; 1997). *Effect of contingency management on adherence to peak flow monitoring in school-age children with asthma* (Doctoral dissertation, University of Pittsburgh, 1996). *Dissertation Abstracts International, 58–01*, 133. (UMI No. 97-18633).

Burroughs, T., Pontious, S., & Santiago, J. (1993). The relationship among six psychosocial domains, age, health care adherence, and metabolic control in adolescents with IDDM. *The Diabetes Educator, 19*(5), 396–402.

Charron-Prochownik, D., Becker, M., Brown, M., Liang, W., & Bennett, S. (1993). Understanding young children's health beliefs and diabetes regimen adherence. *The Diabetes Educator, 19*(5), 409–418.

Christiaanse, M., Lavigne, J., & Lerner, C. (1989). Psychosocial aspects of compliance in children and adolescents with asthma. *Developmental and Behavioral Pediatrics, 10*(2),75–80.

Cohen, B., Kagan, L., Richter, B., Topor, M., & Saveedra, M. (1991). Children's compliance to dialysis. *Pediatric Nursing, 17*(4), 359–365, 420.

Coutts, J., Gibson, N., & Paton, Y. (1992). Measuring compliance with inhaled medication in asthma. *Archives of the Disabled Child, 67*, 332–333.

Creer, T., Backial, M., Burns, K., Leung, P., Marion, R., Miklich, D., Morrill, C., Taplin, P., & Ullman, S. (1988). Living with Asthma: I. Genesis and development of a self-management program for childhood asthma. *Journal of Asthma, 25*(6), 335–362.

D'Angelo, E., Woolf, A., Bessette, J., Rappaport, L., & Ciborowski, J. (1992). *Journal of Clinical Psychology, 48*(5), 672–680.

Daviss, W., Coon, H., Whitehead, P., Ryan, K., Burkley, M., & McMahon, W. (1995). Predicting diabetic control from competence, adherence, adjustment, and psychopathology. *Journal of American Academy of Child & Adolescent Psychiatry, 34*(12), 1629–1636.

Delamater, A., Smith, J., Kurtz, S., & White, N. (1988). Dietary skills and adherence in children with Type I diabetes mellitus. *The Diabetes Educator, 14*(1), 33–36.

Drozda, D., Allen, S., Turner, A., Slusher, J., & McCain, G. (1993). Adherence behaviors in research protocols: Comparison of two interventions. *The Diabetes Educator, 19*(5), 393–395.

Dunbar, J. (1983). Compliance in pediatric populations: A review. In P. McGrath & P. Firestone (Eds.), *Pediatric and adolescent behavioral medicine* (pp. 210–230). New York: Springer.

Dunbar-Jacob, J., Dunning, E., & Dwyer, K. (1993). Compliance research in pediatric and adolescent populations: Two decades of research. In N. Krasnegor, L. Epstein, S. Johnson, & S. Yaffe (Eds.), *Developmental aspects of health compliance behavior* (pp. 29–51). Hillsdale, NJ: Lawrence Erlbaum.

Engel, J. (1993). Children's compliance with progressive relaxation procedures for improving headache control. *The Occupational Therapy Journal of Research, 13*(4), 219–230.

Erikson, E. (1963). *Childhood and society* (2nd ed.). New York: W. W. Norton.

Ferrane, L., & Cox, C. (1993). Determinants of positive health behavior in middle childhood. *Nursing Research, 42*(4), 208–213.

Festa, R., Tamaroff, M., Chasalow, F., & Lanzkowsky, P. (1992). Therapeutic adherence to oral medication regimens by adolescents with cancer: I. Laboratory assessment. *The Journal of Pediatrics, 120*(5), 807–811.

Finney, J., Lemanek, K., Brophy, C., & Cataldo, M. (1990). Pediatric appointment keeping: Improving adherence in a primary care allergy clinic. *Journal of Pediatric Psychology, 15*(4), 571–579.

Foulkes, L., Boggs, S., Fennell, R., & Skibinski, K. (1993). Social support, family variables, and compliance in renal transplant children. *Pediatric Nephrology, 7,* 185–188.

Fraser, J. (1990). Immunization status of chronically ill children. *Texas Medicine/The Journal, 86*(10), 76–79.

Freund, A., Johnson, S., Silverstein, J., & Thomas, J. (1991). Assessing daily management of childhood diabetes using 24-hour recall interviews: Reliability and stability. *Health Psychology, 10*(3), 200–208.

Greenan-Fowler, E., Powell, C., & Varni, J. (1987). Behavioral treatment of adherence to therapeutic exercise by children with hemophilia. *Archives of Physical Medicine & Rehabilitation, 68,* 846–849.

Hanna, K., Ewart, C., & Kwiterovich, P. (1990). Child problem solving competence, behavioral adjustment and adherence to lipid-lowering diet. *Patient Education and Counseling, 16,* 119–131.

Hanson, C., De Guire, M., Schinkel, A., & Henggeler, S. (1992). Comparing social learning and family systems correlates of adaptation in youths with IDDM. *Journal of Pediatric Psychology, 17*(5), 555–572.

Hanson, C., Harris, M., Relyea, G., Cigrang, J., Carle, D., & Burghen, G. (1989). Coping styles of youth with insulin-dependent diabetes mellitus. *Journal of Consulting and Clinical Psychology, 57*(5), 644–651.

Hauser, S., Jacobson, A., Lavori, P., Wolfsdorf, J., Herskowitz, R., Milley, J., & Bliss, R. (1990). Adherence among children and adolescents with insulin-dependent diabetes mellitus over a four-year longitudinal follow-up: II. Immediate and long-term linkages with the family milieu. *Journal of Pediatric Psychology, 15*(4), 527–542.

Haynes, R. (1979). Introduction. In R. Haynes, D. Taylor, & D. Sackett (Eds.), *Compliance in health care* (pp. 1–45). Baltimore, MD: Johns Hopkins University Press.

Hazzard, A., Hutchinson, S., & Krawiecki, N. (1990). Factors related to adherence to medication regimens in pediatric seizure patients. *Journal of Pediatric Psychology, 15*(4), 543–555.

Hentinen, M., & Kyngas, H. (1992). Compliance of young diabetics with health regimens. *Journal of Advanced Nursing, 17*, 530–536.

Hudson, J., Fielding, D., Jones, S., & McKendrick, T. (1987). Adherence to medical regime and related factors in youngsters on dialysis. *British Journal of Clinical Psychology, 26*, 61–62.

Hughes, D., McLeod, M., Garner, B., & Goldbloom, R. (1991). Controlled trial of a home and ambulatory program for asthmatic children. *Pediatrics, 87*(1), 54–61.

Israel, A., Silverman, W., & Solotar, L. (1987). Baseline adherence as a predictor of dropout in a children's weight-reduction program. *Journal of Consulting and Clinical Psychology, 55*(5), 791–793.

Jacobson, A., Hauser, S., Lavori, P., Wolfsdorf, J., Herskowitz, R., Milley, J., Bliss, R., & Gelfand, E. (1990). Adherence among children and adolescents with insulin-dependent diabetes mellitus over a four-year longitudinal follow-up: I. The influence of patient coping and adjustment. *Journal of Pediatric Psychology, 15*(4), 511–526.

Johnson, S., & Kelly, M. (1992). A longitudinal analysis of adherence and health status in childhood diabetes. *Journal of Pediatric Psychology, 17*(5), 537–553.

Johnson, S., Tomer, A., Cunningham, W., & Henretta, J. (1990). Adherence in childhood diabetes: Results of a confirmatory factor analysis. *Health Psychology, 9*(4), 493–501.

Kovacs, M., Goldston, D., Obrosky, S., & Iyengar, S. (1992). Prevalence and predictors of pervasive noncompliance with medical treatment among youths with insulin-dependent diabetes mellitus. *Journal of American Academy of Child & Adolescent Psychiatry, 31*(6), 1112–1119.

Kovacs, M., Charron-Prochownik, D., & Obrosky, D. (1995). A longitudinal study of biomedical and psychosocial predictors of multiple hospitalizations among young people with insulin-dependent diabetes mellitus. *Diabetic Medicine, 12*, 142–148.

La Greca, A., Auslander, W., Greco, P., Spetter, D., Fisher, E., & Santiago, J. (1995). I get by with a little help from my family and friends: Adolescents' support for diabetes care. *Journal of Pediatric Psychology, 20*(4), 449–476.

Lopreiato, J., & Ottolini, M. (1996). Assessment of immunization compliance among children in the department of defense health care system. *Pediatrics, 97*(3), 308–311.

Maiman, L., Becker, M., Liptak, G., Nazarian, L., & Rounds, K. (1988). Improving pediatricians' compliance-enhancing practices. *American Journal of Diseases of Childhood, 142*, 773–779.

Manne, S., Jacobsen, P., Gorfinkle, K., Gerstein, F., & Redd, W. (1993). Treatment adherence difficulties among children with cancer: The role of parenting style. *Journal of Pediatric Psychology, 18*(1), 47–62.

Marteau, T., Johnston, M., Baum, J., & Bloch, S. (1987). Goals of treatment in diabetes: A comparison of doctors and parents of children with diabetes. *Journal of Behavioral Medicine, 10*(1), 33–48.

Miller-Johnson, S., Emery, R., Marvin, R., Clarke, W., Lovinger, R., & Martin, M. (1994). Parent-child relationships and the management of insulin-dependent diabetes mellitus. *Journal of Consulting and Clinical Psychology, 62*(3), 603–610.

National Center for Health Statistics. (1994). *Current estimates from the National Health Interview Survey, 1994* (DHHS Publication No. PHS 96–1521). Washington, DC: U.S. Government Printing Office.

National Center for Health Statistics. (1995). *Current estimates from the National Health Interview Survey, 1994* (Series 10, No. 193). Washington, DC: U.S. Government Printing Office.

Paynter, E., Jordan, W., & Finch, D. (1990). Patient compliance with cleft palate team regimens. *Journal of Speech and Hearing Disorders, 55*, 740–750.

Paynter, E., Wilson, B., & Jordan, W. (1993). Improved patient compliance with cleft palate team regimes. *Cleft Palate-Craniofacial Journal, 30*(3), 292–301.

Phipps, S., & DeCuir-Whalley, S. (1990). Adherence issues in pediatric bone marrow transplantation. *Journal of Pediatric Psychology, 15*(4), 459–475.

Piaget, J. (1951). *Play, dreams, and imitation in childhood.* New York: W. W. Norton.

Piers, E., & Harris, D. (1984). *Piers-Harris Children's Self-Concept Scale.* Los Angeles, CA: Western Psychological Services.

Pinzone, H., Carlson, B., Kotses, H., & Creer, T. (1991). Prediction of asthma episodes in children using peak expiratory flow rates, medication compliance, and exercise data. *Annals of Allergy, 67*, 481–486.

Rapoff, M., Purviance, M., & Lindsley, C. (1988). Educational and behavioral strategies for improving medication compliance in juvenile rheumatoid arthritis. *Archives of Physical Medicine & Rehabilitation, 69*, 439–441.

Reid, G., Dubow, E., Carey, T., & Dura, J. (1994). Contribution of coping to medical adjustment and treatment responsibility among children and adolescents with diabetes. *Developmental and Behavioral Pediatrics, 15*(5), 327–335.

Rotter, J. (1954). *Social learning and clinical psychology.* Englewood Cliffs, NJ: Prentice-Hall.

Schlundt, D., Pichert, J., Rea, M., Puryear, W., Penha, M., & Kline, S. (1994). Situational obstacles to adherence for adolescents with diabetes. *The Diabetes Educator, 20*(3), 207–211.

Schoni, M., Horak, E., & Nikolaizik, W. (1995). Compliance with therapy in children with respiratory diseases. *European Journal of Pediatrics, 154*(Suppl. 3), 77–81.

Szilagyi, P., Rodewald, L., Savageau, J., Yoos, L., & Doane, C. (1992). Improving influenza vaccination rates in children with asthma: A test of a computerized reminder system and an analysis of factors predicting vaccination compliance. *Pediatrics, 90*(6), 871–875.

Taggart, V. S., Zuckerman, A. E., Lucas, S., Acty-Linsey, A., & Bellanti (1987). Adapting a self-management education program for asthma for use in an outpatient clinic. *Annals of Allergy, 58*(3), 173–178.

Tamaroff, M., Festa, R., Adesman, A., & Walco, G. (1992). Therapeutic adherence to oral medication regimens by adolescents with cancer: II. Clinical and psychologic correlates. *The Journal of Pediatrics, 120*(5), 812–817.

U.S. Department of Health and Human Services. (1991). *Healthy people 2000: National health promotion and disease prevention objectives* (DHHS Publication No. PHS 91–50212). Washington, DC: U.S. Government Printing Office.

Weiss, K., Gergen, P., & Hodgson, T. (1992). An economic evaluation of asthma in the United States. *New England Journal of Medicine, 326*(13), 862–866.

Wysocki, T., Hough, B., Ward, K., & Green, L. (1992). Diabetes mellitus in the transition to adulthood: Adjustment, self-care, and health status. *Developmental and Behavioral Pediatrics, 13*(3), 194–201.

Wysocki, T., Taylor, A., Hough, B., Linscheid, T., Yeates, K., & Naglieri, J. (1996). Deviation from developmentally appropriate self-care autonomy. *Diabetes Care, 19*(2), 119–125.

Zora, J., Lutz, C., & Tinkelman, D. (1989). Assessment of compliance in children using inhaled beta adrenergic agonists. *Annals of Allergy, 62*, 406–409.

Index

Springer Publishing Company

Key Aspects of Preventing and Managing Chronic Illness

Sandra G. Funk, PhD, **Elizabeth M. Tornquist,** MA
Jennifer Leeman, DrPH, MDiv, **Margaret S. Miles,** PhD, RN, and
Joanne S. Harrell, PhD, RN, Editors

This latest volume in the award-winning Key Aspects series is a compendium of current research on chronic illness. It includes an overview of important issues in chronic illness—such as self-management and health behavior change—by some of the most distinguished experts in the field. Contributors include Martha Hill, Kate Lorig, and Susan Folkman.

> KEY ASPECTS
> OF
> PREVENTING AND
> MANAGING
> CHRONIC
> ILLNESS
>
> Sandra G. Funk,
> Elizabeth M. Tornquist,
> Jennifer Leeman, Margaret S. Miles,
> and Joanne S. Harrell
> Editors
>
> Springer Publishing Company

Partial Contents

- Chronic Illness: Improving Nursing Practice Through Research
- Closing the Gap Between Information & Action
- Promoting Healthier Behaviors
- Identification of High Risk Adolescents for Interventions to Lower Blood Pressure
- Regular Physical Activity in Older African-Americans
- Early Interventions with Children: A Systems Approach
- Heart Failure: Living With Uncertainty
- Self-Care Decision Making in Clients With Diabetes and Hypertension
- Effects of Exercise on Fatigue: Aerobic Fitness & Disease Activity in Persons With Rheumatoid Arthritis
- Helping Patients With Localized Prostate Cancer: Managing After Treatment
- Patient Knowledge & Self Efficacy for Diabetes Management
- A Survey of Leading Chronic Disease Management Programs
- Coping With Chronic Illness: Lessons From AIDS Caregivers
- Strategies for Using Research to Improve Care

Nurse's Book Society Selection
2001   416pp   0-8261-1352-4   hardcover

536 Broadway, New York, NY 10012 • Telephone: 212-431-4370
Fax: 212-941-7842 • Order Toll-Free: 877-687-7476
Order On-line: www.springerpub.com

Springer Publishing Company

Annual Review of
Nursing Research
Volume 18: Focus on Chronic Illness

Joyce J. Fitzpatrick, PhD, RN, FAAN, Series Editor
Jean Goeppinger, PhD, RN, FAAN, Volume Editor

"★★★★!" "Nowhere else is there such a valuable and important summary of the current research regarding current outcomes for patients with chronic illnesses...motivates the reader to read all chapters and not just the chapter relevant to his or her interest."

—Doody's Publishing, Inc.

This volume addresses the wide-range of chronic illnesses that nurses encounter in their work. The format is the same as previous volumes, with each chapter presenting a careful and systematic review of all available research on specific topics. Important issues in chronic issues are reflected throughout, such as a prolonged and uncertain course of illness, lack of easy resolution, rarity of complete cure, frequent unknown etiology, and multiple risk factors. The book ends with a milestone chapter by Susan Donaldson which overviews significant breakthroughs in nursing research over the past 40 years.

Partial Contents

Part I: Research in Chronic Illness

- What We Know and Don't Know About Chronic Illness Experience

- Interventions for Children with Diabetes and Their Families

- Family Interventions to Prevent Substance Abuse: Children and Adolescents

- Adherence in Chronic Disease

Part II: Milestones in Nursing Research

- Breakthroughs in Scientific Research: The Discipline of Nursing 1960-1999

AJN Book of the Year Award Winner • One of Doody's "250 Best" Books!
2000   344pp   0-8261-1328-1   hardcover

536 Broadway, New York, NY 10012 • Telephone: 212-431-4370
Fax: 212-941-7842 • Order Toll-Free: 877-687-7476
Order On-line: www.springerpub.com